Keto Diet + Anti-Inflammatory Diet + Paleo Diet For Beginners: 3 in 1

Keto Diet For Beginners

Table of Contents

Anti-Inflammatory Diet For Beginners

Table of Contents

Paleo Diet For Beginners

Table of Contents

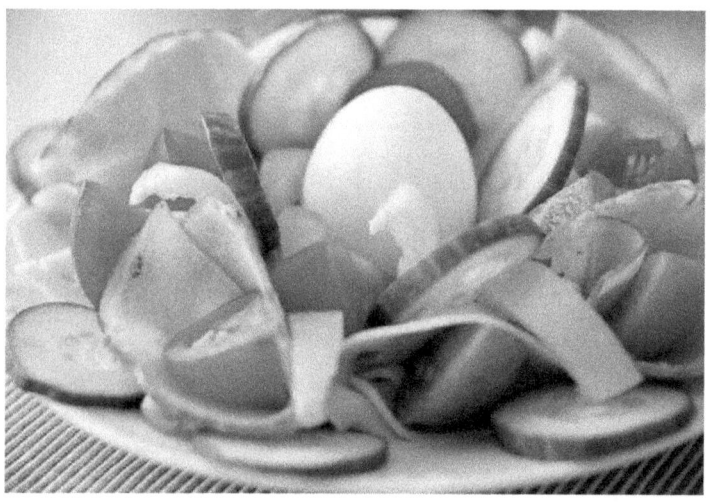

A keto diet is well known for being a low carb diet, where the body produces ketones in the liver to be used as energy. It's referred to as many different names ketogenic diet, low carb diet, low carb high fat (LCHF), etc.

When you eat something high in carbs, your body will produce glucose and insulin.

Glucose is the easiest molecule for your body to convert and use as energy so that it will be chosen over any other energy source.

Insulin is produced to process the glucose in your bloodstream by taking it around the body.

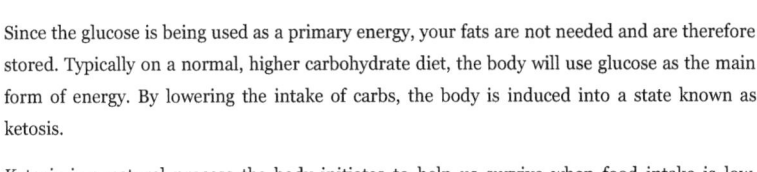

Since the glucose is being used as a primary energy, your fats are not needed and are therefore stored. Typically on a normal, higher carbohydrate diet, the body will use glucose as the main form of energy. By lowering the intake of carbs, the body is induced into a state known as ketosis.

Ketosis is a natural process the body initiates to help us survive when food intake is low. During this state, we produce ketones, which are produced from the breakdown of fats in the liver.

The end goal of a properly maintained keto diet is to force your body into this metabolic state. We don't do this through starvation of calories but starvation of carbohydrates. Reading this Guide will enlight you on the keto diet, stay cool!!

UNDERSTANDING KETOSIS AND KETONES

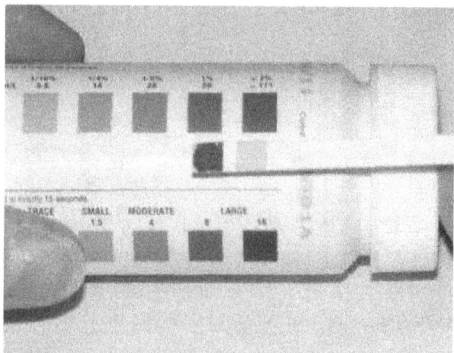

Ketogenic diets are basically designed to induce a state of ketosis in the body. When the amount of glucose in the body becomes too low, the body switches to fat as an alternative source of energy.

The body has two primary fuel sources which are:

Fat deposits are stored in the form of triglycerides. They are normally broken down into long-chain fatty acids and glycerol. Stripping off the glycerol from the triglyceride molecule allows for the release of the three free fatty acid (FFA) molecules into the bloodstream to be used as energy.

The glycerol molecule goes into the liver where three molecules of it combine to form one glucose molecule. Therefore, as your body burns fat, it also produces glucose as a by-product. This glucose can be used to fuel parts of the brain as well as other parts of the body that cannot run on FFA.

However, while glucose can travel through the bloodstream on its own, cholesterol and triglycerides need a carrier to move around in the bloodstream. Cholesterol and triglycerides are packaged in a carrier called low-density lipoprotein, or LDL. Thus, the larger the LDL particle, the more triglycerides it contains.

The overall process of burning fat deposits for energy produces carbon dioxide, water, and compounds called ketones.

Ketones are produced by the liver from free fatty acids. There are composed of 2 groups of atoms linked together by a carbonyl functional group.

The body has no capability to store ketones and therefore they must be either used or excreted. The body excrete them either through the breath as acetone or through the urine as acetoacetate.

Ketones can be used by body cells as a source of energy. Also, the brain can make use of ketones in generating about 70-75% of its energy requirement.

Like alcohol, ketones take priority as a fuel source over carbohydrates. This implies that when they are high in the bloodstream, they must be burned first before glucose can be used as a fuel.

What Causes Ketosis

When you start eating less amounts of carbohydrates, your body gets smaller supply of glucose to use as energy compared to before.

The decrease in the amount of consumed carbohydrates and the subsequent reduction in the amount of available glucose, slowly forces the body to move into the state of ketosis. Thus, the body goes into a state of ketosis when there is not enough amount of glucose available to the body cells.

Starvation Induced Ketosis

Fasting and starvation states usually involve reduced or no intake of food that the body can digest and convert into glucose. While starvation is involuntary, fasting is a more conscious choice you make to intentionally not eat.

However, the body enters into a "starvation mode" whenever you are sleeping, when you skip a meal or when you intentionally go on a fast. The lack of food intake results in a reduction in blood glucose levels. As a result, the body starts to break down it glycogen (stored glucose) stores for energy.

The glycogen is converted back into glucose and used as energy by the body. In this state, the body also starts to burn its stored fats. Thus, the production of ketone bodies (ketogenesis) is induced by a lack of available glucose.

Any time the amount of ketones in the blood outnumber the molecules of glucose, the body cells will start making use of the ketones as their source of energy.

HOW DOES THE KETO DIET WORK

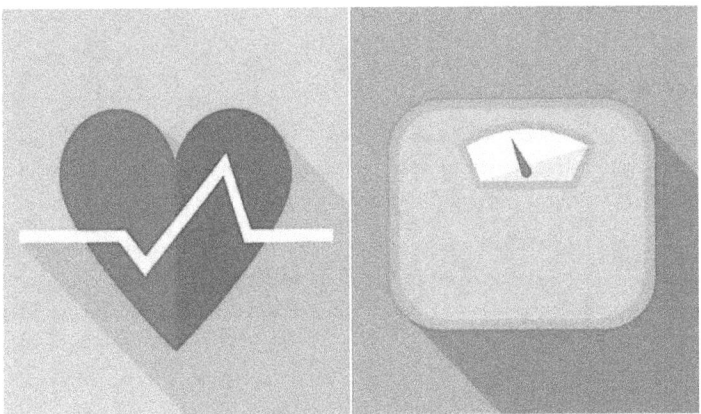

When you eat a diet rich in carbohydrates, your body converts those carbs into glucose (blood sugar). Since carbohydrates are turned into sugar, your blood sugar levels rise.

When blood sugar levels rise, it signals your body to create insulin, which carries glucose to your cells to be used for energy.

Glucose is the preferred energy source of your body. As long as you keep eating carbohydrates, your body will keep turning it into sugar, thereby burning that sugar for energy. In other words, when glucose is present, your body will refuse to burn off its fat stores.

Since carbs are your body's preferred energy source, the only way to start burning fat is by removing carbs.

Cutting carbs depletes your glycogen stores (stored glucose). And with no glucose available for energy, your body has no choice but to start burning its fat stores. Your body starts converting fatty acids into ketones, a metabolic state known as ketosis, and the basis of a ketogenic diet.

What Are Ketones?

In ketosis, your liver converts fatty acids into ketone bodies or ketones. These byproducts become your body's new energy source. When you increase your fat intake, your body responds by becoming "keto-adaptive," or more efficient at burning fat.

Ketosis is a natural survival function of your body. It helps your body function on stored body fat when food is not readily available. Similarly, the keto diet focuses on "starving" your body of carbohydrates, transforming your body into a fat-burning state and supplementing with optimal nutrition.

The three main ketone bodies that your metabolism produces are: Acetoacetate

(AcAc)

Beta-hydroxybutyric acid (BHB) Acetone

The Difference Between Keto, Low-Carb, and Atkins

Too often, the keto diet gets lumped in with other low-carbohydrate diets, like the Atkins Diet. There are a few key differences between them.

Difference In Carbohydrate Intake

The main difference between keto and low-carb is the macronutrient levels. Low-carb diets are considered any diet with a carb intake under about 100-150 grams of carbs per day. It's likely that you'll have to lower your carb intake much more to enter a state of ketosis.

The Atkins Diet is different from keto because of its different phases, which range from severely restricting carbs to adding a liberal amount of carbs (about 80-100 grams daily) back into the diet.

The keto diet works best when you stick to consistently low carb intake under about 50 grams per day for most people.

Difference In Protein Intake

Most low-carb diets are also high-protein diets. However, the keto diet ranges in protein intake, from moderate (around 20% of your total calories) to high-protein intake.

High-protein intake was once thought to spike blood sugar on a ketogenic diet, but there's evidence that you don't need to worry about gluconeogenesis as much as once thought. Still, diets like Atkins depend heavily on protein, without healthy, low-carb veggies for a majority of the diet.

If you're unsure of your optimal protein intake, check out the Keto Calculator to get your unique macronutrient guidelines.

Difference In Goals

The goals between these diets vary as well. The goal of keto is to enter ketosis, weaning your body off burning glucose for fuel for the long-term.

You may never enter ketosis with a low-carb diet. And although you may enter ketosis for a brief period on the Atkins Diet, you'll pop right back out in Phases 3 and 4 as you reintroduce higher levels of carbohydrate-rich foods.

Ketogenic Diet Macronutrients

Macronutrients seem to be the cornerstone of any keto diet, but contrary to popular opinion, there is no ONE macronutrient ratio that works for everyone.

Instead, you're going to have a completely different set of macros than your friend or your mother based on:

Your physical and mental goals Your

health history

Your activity level

The best way to figure these numbers out quickly is to refer to this macronutrient calculator.

Outside of your personal macros, there are general macro guidelines for a ketogenic diet:

70-80% of calories from fats

20-25% of calories from protein

5-10% of calories from carbohydrates

Below, these percentages are broken down into grams. Remember, these should be used as a guideline only. Your macronutrient goals will vary depending on your particular lifestyle.

Fat Intake

Fat is known as the cornerstone of the keto diet because fat does not raise your blood glucose like protein and carbs.

It was once thought that, in order to get into ketosis, you needed to eat massive amounts of fat on a daily basis. However, that's just not true.

The real secret to getting into ketosis is to cut carbs. You can modulate your fat intake from there. However, the accepted rule of thumb for most keto dieters is to stick to anywhere from 70-80% of your calories from healthy fats.

That means, if you're consuming 2,000 calories per day, you would need 144 to 177 grams of fat.

Protein Intake

Protein has gotten a bad rap in the keto community. Some experts claimed that eating too much protein on a very low-carb diet could trigger a metabolic effect called gluconeogenesis.

Protein is extremely important on the keto diet especially if you're active or an athlete.

Ideally, you should consume at least 0.8 grams of protein per pound of lean body mass to prevent muscle loss. For those of you with an extremely active lifestyle, 1 gram of protein per pound of lean body mass is ideal.

To calculate your lean body mass, you have to:

Calculate your body fat percentage. Click here to read how.

Subtract your body fat % from 100%. This will be your lean body mass %.

Multiply your lean body mass % by your total weight.

Or, you can check out the Keto Calculator to figure out your ideal protein intake.

So while most keto sites recommend 10-15% of total calories from protein, know that you can eat a lot more without raising your blood glucose or kicking you out of ketosis.

Carbohydrate Intake

Most people who want to get into ketosis should get about 5-10% of total calories from carbohydrates.

This usually looks like anywhere from 100-200 calories from carbs or about 25-50 grams of carbohydrates per day.

Most people consume roughly 30 grams of carbohydrates on the keto diet. Depending upon your activity level and health needs, you might be able to consume 80 grams of carbs and remain in ketosis.

Different Types of Ketogenic Diets

There are five main approaches to the ketogenic diet. When deciding which method works best for you, take into account your goals, fitness level, and what's realistic for your lifestyle.

The Standard Ketogenic Diet (Skd)

This is the most common and recommended version of the diet. Here, you stay within 20-50 grams of net carbs per day, focusing on moderate protein intake and high fat intake.

Targeted Ketogenic Diet (Tkd)

If you are an active individual, this approach might work best for you. Targeted keto involves eating roughly 25-50 grams of net carbs or less 30 minutes to an hour before exercise.

Cyclical Ketogenic Diet (CKD)

If keto seems intimidating to you, this is an excellent method to start with. You cycle between periods of eating a low-carb diet for several days, followed by a period of eating higher amounts of carbs (typically lasting several days).

High-Protein Ketogenic Diet (Hpkd)

This approach is very similar to the standard (SKD) approach. The primary difference is your protein intake. While a standard keto diet will include moderate protein, here you up your protein intake considerably.

Plant-Based Keto

Plant-based keto could range from eating more low-carb vegetables to going keto as a full-on vegan or vegetarian. You can follow the ketogenic diet as a vegetarian or as a vegan, but it will take a lot of work and effort to do this safely.

What Can You Eat on a Keto Diet?

Now that you understand the basics behind the keto diet, it's time to hit the grocery store.

On the keto diet, you'll enjoy nutrient-dense foods including meat, vegetables, nuts and seeds, and plenty of healthy fats.

You'll also avoid grains, legumes, processed foods, and most fruits. Consume these keto-friendly foods while staying within your macro guidelines:

Meat, Eggs, And Nuts

All meat and seafood are included on the keto diet, as long as they're, not breaded or fried.

Always choose the highest quality meat, you can afford, selecting grass-fed and organic beef whenever possible, wild-caught fish, and pasture-raised poultry, pork, and eggs.

Nuts and seeds are also fine and best eaten raw (not roasted or coated in sugar).

Enjoy:

Beef, preferably fattier cuts like steak, veal, roast, ground beef and stews

Poultry, including chicken breasts, quail, duck, turkey and wild game try to focus on the darker, fattier meats

Pork, including pork loin, tenderloin, chops, ham, and sugar-free bacon

Fish, including mackerel, tuna, salmon, trout, halibut, cod, catfish, and mahi-mahi

Shellfish, including oysters, clams, crab, mussels, and lobster

Organ meats, including heart, liver, tongue, kidney, and offal

Eggs, including deviled, fried, scrambled and boiled use the whole egg Lamb

Goat

Vegetarian sources, like macadamia nuts, almonds, and nut butter

Low-Carb Vegetables

On a keto meal plan, feel free to fill your plate with low-carb vegetables.

Vegetables are a great way to get a healthy dose of micronutrients, thus preventing vitamin deficiencies on keto.

Enjoy low-carb vegetables like leafy greens, and cruciferous veggies, aiming to eat veggies that contain fewer than 5 grams of net carbs per serving.

Enjoy these low carb vegetables:

Leafy greens, such as kale, spinach, swiss chard and arugula Cruciferous

vegetables, including cabbage, cauliflower, and zucchini Lettuces, including

iceberg, romaine, and butterhead

Fermented vegetables like sauerkraut and kimchi

Other vegetables such as mushrooms, asparagus, and celery

Keto-Friendly Dairy

If you can tolerate dairy, it is allowed on the keto diet. Choose the highest quality you can reasonably afford, selecting grass-fed, whole-fat, and organic dairy whenever possible.

Keto-friendly dairy options include: Butter

and ghee

Heavy cream and heavy whipping cream Fermented

dairy products like yogurts and kefir Sour cream

Hard and soft cheeses

Low-Sugar Fruits

Approach fruit with caution on keto, as it contains high amounts of sugar and carbohydrates. If you are craving something light and sweet, grab a handful of berries, such as blueberries or raspberries, as a treat.

Enjoy these low sugar fruits:

Avocadoes (the one fruit you can enjoy in abundance)

Organic berries, such as raspberries, blueberries, strawberries, and cranberries

Healthy Fats And Oils

You can enjoy both animal fats (saturated fats) and plant-based fats on a healthy keto diet.

Healthy fat sources include grass-fed butter, tallow, and ghee or coconut oil, olive oil, sustainable palm oil and MCT oil from plants.

Enjoy these fats and oils on keto: Butter

and ghee

Lard Mayonnaise

Coconut oil, coconut butter

Flaxseed oil

Olive oil Sesame seed

oil

MCT oil and MCT powder

Walnut oil

Olive oil, avocado oil

Herbs And Spices

Use seasonings freely on keto just make sure they don't have any added sugar. To add

flavor to dishes, consider purchasing fresh herbs at the store.

Pro tip: If you store fresh herbs in a mason jar filled with water in the fridge, they will last up to two weeks.

Foods to Avoid on a Keto Diet

It's best to avoid the following foods on a keto diet due to their high carb content.

When starting keto, do a purge of your fridge and cupboards. Donate any unopened items and throw the rest away.

Grains

Grains are loaded with carbs, so it's best to avoid all grains on keto. Whole grains, wheat, pasta, rice, oats, barley, rye, corn, and quinoa are all out. Instead, try one of these substitutes.

Beans And Legumes

While many vegans and vegetarians rely beans for their protein content, they are actually incredibly high-carb. Avoid eating kidney beans, chickpeas, black beans, and lentils.

Higher-Sugar Fruits

While many fruits are packed with antioxidants and other micronutrients, they're also high in fructose, which will kick you out of ketosis.

Avoid apples, mangos, pineapple and other fruits (with the exception of small amounts of berries).

Starchy Veggies

Avoid starchy vegetables like potatoes, sweet potatoes, some squash, parsnips, and carrots.

Like fruit, there are health benefits to these foods. However, you can find those vitamins and minerals from low-carb sources ones that won't kick you out of ketosis.

Sugar

This includes, but is not limited to desserts, artificial sweeteners, smoothies, soda, and fruit juice.

Even condiments like ketchup and BBQ sauce are usually filled with sugar, so put down the ketchup bottle. If you are craving a dessert, try one of these keto-friendly recipes instead.

Alcohol

Some alcoholic beverages are low-glycemic and appropriate for a ketogenic diet. However, keep in mind that when you drink alcohol, your liver will preferentially process the ethynol and stop producing ketones.

If you're on a ketogenic diet to lose weight, keep your alcohol consumption to a minimum. If you're craving a cocktail, stick to low-sugar mixers and avoid most beer and wine.

Seed Oils

Seed oils are heavily processed and can become oxidized (aka, rancid) when you heat them. Avoid corn oil, canola oil, peanut oil, and grapeseed oil. They also contain large amounts of omega–6 fatty acids, which are inflammatory in large amounts.

Health Benefits of a Keto Diet

A ketogenic diet has been associated with incredible health benefits that stretch way beyond weight loss. Here are just a few ways keto may help you feel better, stronger, and more clear-headed:

Keto For Weight Loss

Probably what the keto diet is most famous for: sustainable fat loss. Keto can significantly decrease body weight, body fat, and body mass while maintaining muscle mass. Keto can also increase fat metabolism during exercise, making it an excellent part of your active lifestyle.

Keto For Endurance Levels

The ketogenic diet may help improve endurance levels for athletes. However, it may take time for athletes to adjust to burning fat instead of glucose for energy.

Keto For Gut Health

Several studies have shown a link between low sugar intake and improvement in symptoms of irritable bowel syndrome (IBS). In fact, one study showed that eating a ketogenic diet can improve abdominal pain and overall quality of life in those with IBS.

Keto For Diabetes

The ketogenic diet helps to balance blood sugar and insulin levels, which helps immensely with metabolic diseases like type 2 diabetes.

Keto For Heart Health

The keto diet can help reduce risk factors for heart disease, including improvement in HDL cholesterol, triglycerides, and LDL cholesterol (related to plaque in the arteries).

Keto For Brain Health

The keto diet may support those with Parkinson's, Alzheimer's disease, and other degenerative brain diseases This is likely because ketone bodies having possible neuroprotective and anti-inflammatory benefits.

Keto For Skin Health

Because ketones and lower blood sugar contribute to overall hormone balance and lower inflammatory markers, the keto diet may be good for skin health. One study suggests that decreased skin inflammation can decrease acne and other skin lesions.

Keto For Epilepsy

The ketogenic diet was created in the early 20th century to help prevent seizures in epileptic patients, especially children. To this day, ketosis is a go-to therapeutic diet for those who suffer from epilepsy.

Keto For Cancer Support

There's a growing body of research that suggests a strict keto diet can help slow tumor growth. Although no one diet can cure or prevent cancer, a low-carb, zero-sugar diet is a great place to start.

Keto For Pms

An estimated 90% of women experience one or more of symptoms associated with PMS. A keto diet can help balance blood sugar, combat chronic inflammation, boost your nutrient stores, and crush cravings all of which may help alleviate your PMS symptoms.

How to Know When You're in Ketosis

You can follow the above macronutrient guidelines, eat the prescribed keto diet foods and avoid grains, starches, and legumes and still struggle to enter ketosis.

Why? Because ketosis is a metabolic state, and you may need to tweak your meal plan, exercise regimen, and other lifestyle choices in order to enter it.

There are plenty of signs and symptoms to suggest you're in ketosis, including: Weight

loss

Fewer cravings Better

mental clarity More stable

energy

But there's only one reliable way to know whether or not you're in ketosis: Test your ketone levels.

There are three ways to do this: In your

urine with a urine strip

In your blood with a glucose meter On your

breath with a breath meter

The Ketogenic Diet Heirarchy of Needs Testing

Each method has its advantages and disadvantages, with a blood test being the most accurate (but most expensive). Although it's the most affordable, urine testing is typically the least accurate method.

Supplements to Support a Keto Diet

Supplements are a popular way to maximize the benefits of a ketogenic diet. You can't get all of your nutrients from supplements and expect to feel good, but they can help.

Add in these supplements alongside a healthy, whole-food based keto diet for the best results.

Exogenous Ketones

"Exogenous ketones" are supplemental ketones usually beta-hydroxybutyrate or acetoacetate that help kick you into ketosis and give you the energy you need to thrive. You can take exogenous ketones in between meals or for a quick burst of energy before a workout.

MCT Oil And Powder

MCTs (or medium-chain triglycerides) are a type of fatty acid that your body can convert to energy quickly and efficiently. Benefits includes weight loss and energy, among other things. MCTs come from coconuts and are sold mostly in liquid form. Perfect Keto sells them as a delicious and easy-to-use powder.

Collagen Protein

Collagen is the most abundant protein in your body, accounting for about 25-35%. It's the glue that holds your body together as it supports the growth of joints, organs, hair, and connective tissues. Amino acids from collagen supplements may also help with energy production, DNA repair, detox, and healthy digestion.

Micronutrient Supplements

It's tough to get all the micronutrients you need from diet alone regardless of what nutrition regimen you're on. Keto Micro Greens is the solution to getting all your micronutrients in one convenient scoop.

Ketogenic Pre-Workout Supplements

Keto pre-workout supplements like Perfect Keto Perform Pre-Workout can boost physical and cognitive performance without the caffeine crash. It contains exogenous ketones and MCT oil powder for energy, creatine for protein metabolism, branched- chain amino acids for muscle growth and repair, and more.

Whey Protein

One of the best-studied supplements for weight loss support, muscle gain and maintenance, and recovery. Make sure to choose grass-fed whey only and avoid powders with sugar or any other additives that could spike blood sugar.

Electrolytes

Electrolyte balance is one of the most critical yet most overlooked components of a successful ketogenic diet experience. Especially when you're just starting out. A keto diet can make you excrete more electrolytes than usual so you have to replenish them yourself. Add more sodium, potassium, and calcium to your diet or grab a supplement that can help.

Krill Oil

Get even more of the benefits of an anti-inflammatory keto diet with some high-quality omega-3 fatty acids. Krill oil is just as potent as fish oil, without the fishy aftertaste. Krill also contains phospholipids and a potent antioxidant called astaxanthin that fish oil doesn't.

Blood Sugar Support

Think about adding vitamins, minerals, and herbs to support normal digestion, metabolism, hormone function, and energy production. Take these with higher carb meals to support healthy carbohydrate metabolism or just to promote healthy nutrient absorption.

Is the Ketogenic Diet Safe?

Ketosis is a perfectly safe and natural metabolic state, but it is often confused with a highly dangerous metabolic state called ketoacidosis.

Having ketone levels in the 0.5-5.0mmol/L range is not dangerous, but other risks include a range of issues, from harmless keto flu symptoms to diabetic ketoacidosis, which is not a problem unless you're diabetic.

Ketoacidosis

Diabetic ketoacidosis (DKA) is a dangerous metabolic state that is most commonly seen in people with type 1 diabetes and sometimes type 2 diabetics if they aren't properly managing their insulin and diet.

Keto Flu Symptoms

Many people deal with common side effects similar to flu-like symptoms as they become fat adapted after decades of running on carbs. These temporary symptoms are byproducts of dehydration and low carbohydrate levels while your body adjusts:

Headaches

Lethargy Nausea

Brain fog

Stomach pain Low

motivation

The keto flu can often be shortened or avoided completely by taking one of our ketone supplements, which help switch the body into ketosis instantly. They make the transition period much shorter and easier.

Different Types of Ketogenic Diets

Over the past several years, people have found different ways to approach the ketogenic diet.

Depending on your goals and fitness level, you may find one type of keto diet fits your lifestyle better than others. No matter which one you choose, the goal should be to shift your body from using carbs to using fat as your primary source of fuel.

Here's a breakdown of the different type of keto diets:

Standard Ketogenic Diet (Skd)

This is the most straightforward approach to the ketogenic diet. On the SKD, you're keeping your total carbs extremely low while focusing most of your macronutrient intake on fat and protein. The goal of SKD is to get into and maintain a state of ketosis, burning fat as your primary source of fuel.

Cyclical Ketogenic Diet (CKD)

The cyclical ketogenic diet is a good choice if your goal is to increase muscle strength and improve exercise performance. When following the CKD you're cycling days of ketosis with days of higher carb intake. A typical CKD will be five to six days eating a keto diet (very low-carb), with one or two days of higher carb intake.

The purpose is to reap the benefits of keto during the days on, and on the re-feeding carb days to restore your glycogen stores for huge amounts of activity.

As mentioned earlier, glucose from carbs is a very readily available source of fuel. For athletes and bodybuilders, this can be a great way to get the best of both worlds.

Targeted Ketogenic Diet(Tkd)

The TKD is similar to the standard ketogenic diet, with the exception that you can eat carbohydrates around (before or after) heavy workouts. This approach is for you if you're performing high-intensity workouts for extended periods of time.

If you exercise regularly and are burning fuel at a significant rate, this may be a good strategy for you. Especially if you find yourself "bonking" during workouts when you're in ketosis.

Some athletes notice a decrease in stamina after they've switched to keto.

This approach allows them to benefit from the rapid fuel source of glucose, while also burning it up quickly enough to get back into a ketogenic state. This strategy is best for people who are working out for an hour or more at a moderate to high intensity.

High-Protein Ketogenic Diet

The high-protein keto diet is becoming popular as more people are discovering that they can eat higher protein while still maintaining a ketogenic state.

A high-protein ketogenic diet should be around 30-35% protein, with 60% fat, keeping carbs just as low as you would on a standard ketogenic diet.

This is a good option for people who are active and want to maintain muscle mass. It's also an approach to play with if you're having a hard time sticking to a very high-fat, low- to moderate-protein diet.

Regardless of your macronutrient ratio, the goal is to maintain a ketogenic state for as much of the time as possible, so you can reap all the benefits of being in a ketogenic state.

Benefits of a Keto Diet

Many anecdotal accounts of the keto diet claim rapid weight loss, better brain function, and fewer food cravings. But there are plenty of scientifically-backed benefits of the keto diet as well. Here are just a few:

Blood Sugar Control

Studies have found that people with type 2 diabetes do exceptionally well on a ketogenic diet. Studies show that the extreme reduction in carbs showed an increase in blood glucose control as well as a reduced need for insulin controlling medication.

Fat Loss

Despite higher caloric intake, the ketogenic diet is superior to a low-fat diet for fat loss. Fat loss around the midsection (metabolically active fat) seems to be a specific target in ketogenic fat loss.

Mental Clarity

Many people report feeling enhanced mental sharpness and clarity when following a ketogenic diet. Part of this response may come from higher energy utilization along with the anti-inflammatory effect of the ketogenic diet.

Blood Lipid Profile

Following a ketogenic diet can improve your blood lipid profile. Specifically, it can increase HDL (good cholesterol) and also increase the size of your LDL particles. Larger, fluffier LDL particles are safer because they are less likely to contribute to plaques.

Lower Inflammation

One of the three ketone bodies, beta-hydroxybutyrate (BHB), has been shown to decrease inflammation in your body by blocking an inflammatory signaling pathway.

Heart Disease

Due to its positive effect on both blood lipids and inflammation, the ketogenic diet may benefit those with or at risk for heart disease.

Neurological Disease

The ketogenic diet has been used for over 80 years to treat epilepsy, a disorder in which the nerve cell activity in your brain is disturbed, leading to seizures.

14 DAY KETO DIET MENU FOR BEGINNERS

WEEK 1:
MONDAY
Breakfast: Cheesy Keto Bagels
Lunch: Zesty Chili Lime Keto Tuna Salad
Dinner: Nutritious Baked Pork Chops

TUESDAY
Breakfast: Avocado Egg Bowls
Lunch: Low-Carb Romanesco with Cabbage Noodles
Dinner: One-Pan Cheesy Broccoli Chicken Casserole
WEDNESDAY
Breakfast: Breakfast Casserole with Bacon, Egg, and Cheese Lunch:
Grass-Fed Keto Beef Bulgogi
Dinner: Lemon Balsamic Chicken

THURSDAY
Breakfast: Cinnamon Dolce Latte Breakfast Smoothie Lunch: Spicy
Ginger Salmon Buddha Bowl
Dinner: Loaded Cauliflower Bake

FRIDAY
Breakfast: Almond Flour Low-Carb Crepes Lunch:
Crispy Parmesan Crusted Chicken
Dinner: Crispy Skin Salmon With Pesto Cauliflower Rice

SATURDAY
Breakfast: Savory Breakfast Keto Sausage Balls Lunch:
Portobello Bun Cheeseburgers
Dinner: Keto Chicken Cordon Blue

SUNDAY
Breakfast: Chocolate Protein Pancakes Lunch:
Keto Low-Carb Chili
Dinner: Stuffed Keto Pork Loin

WEEK 2: MONDAY
Breakfast: Keto N'oatmeal
Lunch: Spicy Low-Carb Salmon Patties
Dinner: Low-Carb Keto Pot Roast

TUESDAY
Breakfast: Turkey Sausage Frittata
Lunch: Rich and Creamy Keto Broccoli Cheese Soup Dinner: Spicy
Grass-Fed Keto Fajitas

WEDNESDAY
Breakfast: Smoked Salmon Keto Avocado Toast Lunch:
Easy Keto Chicken Salad
Dinner: Keto Grass-Fed Beef Stew

THURSDAY
Breakfast: Pumpkin Cream Cheese Muffins Lunch:
Zesty Keto Taco Salad
Dinner: Tender Keto Pork Chops

FRIDAY
Breakfast: Micronutrient Greens Matcha Smoothie Lunch:
Curry Chicken Lettuce Wraps
Dinner: Fathead Pizza: Low-Carb Keto Pizza

SATURDAY
Breakfast: Keto Egg Muffins
Lunch: Low-Carb Cauliflower Mac and Cheese Dinner:
Delicious Low-Carb Keto Meatloaf

SUNDAY
Breakfast: Fluffy Salted Caramel Pumpkin Spice Pancakes Lunch:
Savory Shrimp Keto Stir-Fry
Dinner: Low-Carb Keto Lasagna

Dessert Options:
Indulgent Keto Peanut Butter Cups
Creamy Chocolate No Churn Keto Ice Cream Thick
and Rich Keto Whipped Cream Matcha Chia Seed
Pudding
Chocolate Sea Salt Peanut Butter Bites
Rich and Creamy Pumpkin Spice Keto Mocha

PROS AND CONS OF KETOGENIC DIETING

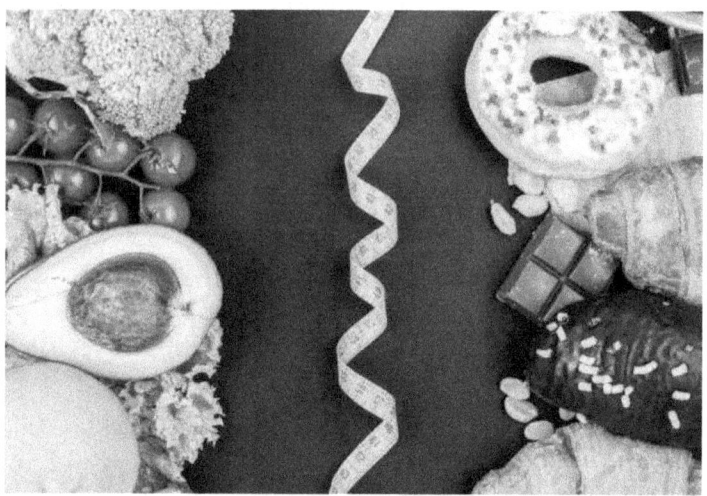

The Atkins diet itself is only the most popular of an approach usually called low-carb diets because of the primary interest in restricting consumption of Carbohydrates. Since the entire spectrum of our food is drawn from proteins, fats, carbohydrates or water, severe restriction of one group is seen by many as an arbitrary and possibly even dangerous step.

Most of the controversy surrounding low-carb approaches is not that they lie about weight-loss (studies continue to show marked weight-loss in many who use the diets) but the disturbing possibility that cutting the carbs out of your diet just isn't healthy. After all, what good is a diet that slims you down only to clog up your arteries and kill you? We've heard many arguments both for and against the use of low-carbohydrate diets, this article asks a radical question: Can going Low-Carb actually be healthy?

Why Should I Limit Sugar & Grains?

The first and most obvious carbohydrate group and one we rarely have much argument about reducing is sugar. Sugar is a catch all term for a number of simple carbohydrates including fructose (fruit sugar), Galactose (milk sugar), sucrose (table sugar) and glucose (simple sugars such as blood sugar). Sugar consumption has been on the increase for decades and, despite the numerous campaigns against saturated fats, is certainly the biggest contributing factor to the increasing obesity epidemic.

Eating sugar causes a number of physiological effects in the body. The most striking of these is the sudden and marked increase in blood insulin. Insulin is the hormone in our body responsible for 'taxiing' the food broken down in out stomach to the various parts of our body that require these substances, although it has numerous uses. First, and most importantly, sugar, as glucose levels in out blood is extremely toxic. Left in our bloodstream without control elevated sugar levels would kill us quickly, so the powerful release of insulin helps keep our blood cleared of excess glucose. Unfortunately insulin is a double-edged sword. Excess sugar in our body cannot be disposed of in an unlimited number of ways. With our increasing sedentary lifestyles refusing to burn off much of this sudden and quick release of carbohydrate as we consume, sugar is rapidly converted to the same saturated fats we are constantly warned about. (As you can see, limiting saturated fat in the diet does not prevent us from accumulating fat in our bodies).

Sugar has other unpleasant side effects. The constantly elevated insulin levels can eventually lead to decreased insulin sensitivity (Syndrome X) and another case of Type II diabetes. Sugar also has an effect on cortisol and our adrenal glands. It causes an excess of these hormones leading to symptoms of stress and fatigue. Sugar also competes with the glucose carriers in our blood, which work with vitamins like Vitamin C, causing disruption to our preciously balanced immune system and causing premature ageing of the skin.

Sugar can be thought of as nitro-fuel for the body. It releases a very quick but harsh burst of artificial energy. Inactive individuals requiring peak performance from athletic pursuits, simple carbohydrates can be a useful tool, especially in the area of pre and post workout drinks. Much like a drag-racer using nitro fuel, this substance can be used to replace muscle glycogen and spare muscle wastage due to overtraining effects. Unfortunately few of us use sugar in this careful and controlled manner and are attempting to drive the finely balanced engines of our bodies on a fuel which causes too much stress and strain on a system that was never designed to handle the excess we provide.

So since low-carb diets almost completely eliminate sugar from our diets, we have already found one significant health benefit.

Grain Controversy

Most of our Western Governments offer health guidelines which ask us to base our food intake almost universally around grain-type carbohydrates, what were once grouped as starches. We know these most commonly as rice, pasta, potatoes and breads. These types of food appear to have been staples of our western diets since time immemorial (they're not, but that's another story). We are often told that eating these foods will leave us full, satisfied and full of a slow releasing stream of energy that is healthy and safe. Unfortunately, at least for human beings, this doesn't always appear to be the case.

Not all grains are created equal for a start and this can be where grain advocates purposely or accidentally mislead. For instance most rice, particularly white rice, will convert to sugar almost immediately in our system and we've already seen some of the devastating effects of excess sugar consumption. Grains, no matter what source they come from will cause elevated insulin levels. For the very healthy amongst us, who have extremely sensitive insulin (either through good genetics, regular exercise or a combination of both) may be able to carefully use small quantities of grains to fuel their bodies through the periods of high activity. However for the vast majority of people, the excess of grains will result in almost all the same problems as sugar consumption. Many low-carb exponents are suspicious of medical advice to eat grains, many citing

Government subsidies of mass agriculture. Eating grains is a very cheap and simple way of providing food, but cheap and simple is rarely the same as healthy and good.

Vegetables!

Low carb diets have often been seen as lacking in vegetables as people carefully trim away all excess carbohydrates, effectively throwing the baby out with the dirty bathwater. On the subject of vegetables, you won't find much dissension amongst medical experts of any standpoint. These wonderful foodstuffs not only contain a plethora of vitamins and minerals, but also are often chock-full of fiber, water and a host of exotic cancer-fighting substances unique to vegetables.

The important thing about vegetables are is that they are nutrient dense and calorie sparse. In plain English, they contain a lot of good stuff in a very small package. You can eat virtually enough vegetables to fill you up and still have eaten only a tiny percentage of the calories a normal diet would confer.

One of the arguments for regular grain consumption is the necessary vitamins and minerals they contain, not to mention the essential fibre for our digestive tract. But guess what? Vegetables makes grains seem pretty redundant. A small handful of organic vegetables will contain more vitamins and minerals than virtually a day's worth of grains, all in an easier to digest package, with extra water and no danger of insulin overload.

Even on a low-carb diet you can stuff yourself silly with vegetables without fear. The primary advantage of a low-carb diet is insulin control and vegetables won't interfere with that. Remember organic vegetables have a much higher vitamin and mineral content, also the darker green or red a vegetable the higher the amount of beneficial Chlorophyll inside the plant. Try to eat your veggies raw and fresh and often. A regular supply of varied veggies is like nature's most perfect multivitamin pill.

Eat Veggies But

What About All The Other Foods You Need?

So low-carb dieters are shedding the pounds by avoiding the insulin spiking grains and sugars. In the process they're moving over to eating other stuff though right? You stop eating bread and pasta and you've got to eat something! We see Atkins dieters especially loading up proteins and fats, burgers, sausages, bacon, full double cream, fried eggs and a host of other tasty but controversial foods. So, fine, we can accept that somehow these people still seem to shed weight much faster and more consistently than their carbohydrate munching friends but surely, surely, that can't be HEALTHY?

Too good to be true? Some Doctors definitely believe so. We've been warned about saturated fat and our rising cholesterol problem for a number of years. Suddenly a diet comes along that seems to throw all that conventional wisdom out of the window.

As it happens, the American Medical Association was forced to declare the Atkins diet 'heart-healthy' after a number of university studies came up with the surprising findings that Atkins dieters were actually lowering their blood fat deposits and sparing the hearts much more than those on a regular higher carb diet.

First we know the basis of that diet is our good friend, the organic vegetable. But moving on, it seems our bodies were designed for a much greater range of essential nutrients than those found in vegetable alone. First up Fats. Yes, it may have finally begun to infiltrate the mainstream press but its old news to many of us. Fat is essential! We need to eat fat. There's no getting around it, our bodies don't merely tolerate the stuff, they absolutely need it to function. When you remember that our brains are over sixty percent fat, our organs require it and our very nerves are built from it, you begin to see how important it is. However much like our friend the Carbohydrate, all fats are not created equal either. Our bodies need a small group of fats that we call 'Essential Fatty Acids'. Our body cannot produce these from any other substances and needs a regular supply or it begins to see shortcomings in its internal workings. We can get by for a while on diminished supplies but our health begins to suffer greatly in the long run.

These healthy fats come in the form of the well-publicised fish and cod-liver oils, flax and various other nut oils and foods like avocado. (Although not essential organic coconut oil has a host of special benefits) Simply be ensuring that a large percentage of our daily fat intake comes from clean, healthy oils will go a long way to improving our health, from defending our brain against degenerative diseases to protecting our skin from the harmful rays of the sun. To be a healthy low carber you need to investigate healthy fats a little more and remember that high quality, preferably organic oils are a better choice than others. There are a host of books on this subject and a host of great products out there. Unfortunately due to the mass pollution of the seas, fish may no longer be the healthiest option, although carefully filtrated fish-oils (by Companies who are clued up on the science of keeping these oils in a health-giving state) are widely available and a must-buy for everyone.

Protein covers the widest range of foods left to us. Protein, which makes up our body's muscles, can be found from the flesh of other animals as well as from milks, beans and lentils. Much like fat, our body requires protein. How much is open to debate. Active individuals, particularly those who require larger muscles, will have a much higher protein need than a sedentary individual but sufficed to say, excess protein intake (although feared by many mainstream nutritionists) has none of the dangers that excess grain or sugar consumption does.

That said, we could always make healthier choices. Although the Atkins diet may allow us to eat burgers and bacon all day long, this may not be the ideal choice. When considering meat products we have to remember what state the animal it came from was in when it was slaughtered. Most animals in large factory farming business are over-fed, over medicated cripples and surely this meat can't be entirely healthy. Foods like bacon also contain a large number of hazardous preservative chemicals that sap at our besieged immune systems. Once again, not all proteins are created equal. Choosing organic fresh meats from leaner animals is a wise choice when considering health.

Chicken and Turkey, from good organic sources is a lean and easy to use protein source. Animals such as bison (buffalo) and Ostrich may sound like exotic food sources to many, but their meat is almost entirely free from chemicals and their natural diets of grass and other non-artificial feeds leaves them with a low-fat content of good, healthy fats. High quality protein is essential to your health and survival. Eating lower-quality meats may allow you to stay trim (since protein consumption appears to regulate our appetite much better than grains ever could) but investing in higher quality meats will mean you can claim the health benefits as well.

The Healthy Low Carb Approach

As many low-carb dieters have pointed out, most humans were never designed to live on a high carbohydrate content in their diets. As hunter-gatherers we consisted mostly on animals that roamed wild and on fresh vegetables and berries we could find in our local habitat. Although our societies may have advanced enough to let us devise sustained agriculture, our genes are still locked in a hundred thousand-year-old struggle for survival. Our bodies recognise the nutrients available from clean meats, healthy fats and fresh vegetables. They have substantial trouble coping with the sudden influx of excess energy and too quickly absorbed carbohydrates in the form of grains and sugars.

Restricting the intake of grains and sugars makes a fairly quick and positive change towards a healthier life. However, it may be that, in our urge to shed the pounds with as little pain as possible, the lower carb diets we choose are tilted towards the proteins and fats we don't really need and attention to vegetables is ignored. With a few minor modifications we can find a lower-carbohydrate approach that not only helps us maintain a normalised body-weight and fat mass but also helps us be an all round healthier individual. There are a hundred other points towards improving health but all these changes make an admirable start.

KETOSIS SIDE EFFECTS

There are many awesome benefits with come with adopting a low-carb ketogenic diet, such as weight loss, decreased cravings, and even possibly reduce diseases risks. That being said, it's also good to talk about possible ketosis side effects so you know fully what to expect as you start this new health journey.

Common Ketosis Side Effects and Treatments

Not everyone experiences side effects when starting a ketogenic diet, and thankfully, those who do don't usually experience them for very long. It varies with the individual, but just to make sure all your bases are covered, we're going to breaking down each possible side effect and go over ways to manage and alleviate them if needed.

- -- FREQUENT URINATION

As your body burns through the stored glucose in your liver and muscles within the first day or two of starting a ketogenic diet, you'll be releasing a lot of water in the process. Plus, your kidneys will start excreting excess sodium as the levels of your circulating insulin drop.

Basically, you might notice yourself needing to pee more often throughout the day. But no worries; this side effect of ketosis takes care of itself once your body adjusts and is no longer burning through the extra glycogen.

- -- DIZZINESS AND DROWSINESS

As the body is getting rid of this excess water, it will also be eliminating minerals like potassium, magnesium, and sodium too. This can make you feel dizzy, lightheaded, and fatigued.

Thankfully, this is also very avoidable; all it takes is a little preparation beforehand. Focus on eating foods that are rich in potassium, such as:

Leafy greens (aim for at least two cups each day!)

Broccoli

Dairy

Meat, poultry, and fish

Avocados

Add salt to your foods or use salty broth when cooking too. You can also dissolve about a teaspoon of regular salt in a glass of water and increase your hydration at the same time.

Adding salt to food might be new to you, since most people are used to being told to limit salt intake. However, when you're eating a ketogenic diet of less than 60 carbohydrates each day, you'll need to make up for this loss of salt. That being said, those with high blood pressure who take medication should check with their doctors before making a change.

- – LOW BLOOD SUGAR

Also known as hypoglycemia, low blood sugar is another common ketosis side effect when beginning a ketogenic diet, especially for people who were used to eating higher amounts of carbs each day. When your body is used to intaking more carbs, it becomes accustomed to putting a certain amount of insulin out to handle the sugar.

So, when the amount of sugar intake is drastically reduced on a keto diet, it's possible to experience short-term episodes of low blood sugar. That can make you feel temporarily tired, hungry, or shaky until your body adjusts.

– – CRAVINGS FOR SUGAR

A great long-term benefit of the ketogenic diet is reduced cravings for sugar and other unhealthy foods. However, you might initially have stronger cravings for carbs during the transition period. This can last anywhere from one to two days to around three weeks. But stick it out! At the end, you'll be pleased with the reduced, and often eliminated, cravings.

– – CONSTIPATION

As your digestive system adapts, you might initially experience some constipation when new to the keto diet. This is often caused by dehydration as you release more fluids (remember how we talked about going to the bathroom more?).

Remedy constipation by making sure your intake of fiber is high, eating tons of non- starchy vegetables, getting enough salt, and drink tons of water each day to moisten the contents of the colon.

If that doesn't help completely, try cutting back on your nut and dairy consumption. You might also consider taking 400 mg of magnesium citrate.

– – DIARRHEA

On the flip side of the previously mentioned side effect, some people might experience minor issues with diarrhea in the first few days. This can simply be a result of your body adjusting to the macronutrient ratio change. In other cases, some people make the mistake of limiting their fat intake along with their carbs, which makes your intake of protein too high and can lead to diarrhea.

Don't skip on your fats! Be sure the carbs you're limiting are being replaced by full fat sources instead of proteins.

– – MUSCLE CRAMPS

Loss of minerals when first starting the keto diet can cause muscle cramps, especially leg cramps, in some people. Like with other side effects we've mentioned, drinking lots of water and eating salt can help by preventing cramps and reducing mineral loss.

– – FLU-LIKE SYMPTOMS

Within the first 2-4 days of beginning a keto diet, a common side effect is known as the "ketosis flu" or "induction flu" because it mimics the symptoms of an actual flu. This means you might experience:

Headaches

Tiredness or lack of motivation

Lethargy

Brain fog or confusion

Irritability

Although these symptoms typically go away completely within a few days, they are also completely avoidable if you stay very hydrated and increase your salt intake (seeing a pattern here?). And like always, be sure you're eating enough fat.

– – SLEEP ISSUES

Some people have reported having trouble sleeping after beginning a ketogenic diet. If this sounds like you, it could mean your serotonin and insulin levels are low.

Try having a snack right before you go to bed that contains protein as well as some carbs to increase insulin and give your brain a nice dose of tryptophan, which is the precursor for serotonin, from the protein.

Another possible reason for impaired sleep could be increased intake of food rich in histamines, which can cause more anxiety and sleeplessness in some people. You can remedy this by eating less cheeses, avocado, bacon, and eggs, which contain a lot of histamines, and replacing them with more vegetables in your diet.

- – SMELLY BREATH

Some people experience the smell of acetone on their breath when eating very low carb. Acetone is one of the ketone bodies created during ketosis, and it has a characteristically fruity smell similar to nail polish remover. This is a sign your body is in ketosis, burning lots of fats and converting them to ketones for energy. That's great news!

Plus, those who notice this smell on their breath or body (and not everyone does) report it usually going away within 1-2 weeks as the body adapts to ketosis. But if it doesn't completely go away in this amount of time, here are some tips for resolving it:

Keep good oral hygiene. Keep your breath fresh by brushing your teeth well at least twice day (hopefully you're doing this already!).

Increase water intake. Bad breath can be caused by less saliva from dry mouth as your body releases water in a low-carb state. Drinking plenty of water will help counteract this.

Use breath freshener. Although this won't eliminate the fruity smell completely, it will mask it as you wait for it to subside.

Slightly increase carbs. If you wait a few more weeks and still have trouble with the ketone smell, you might consider eating slightly more carbs to reduce the ketosis. Try increasing to between 50 and 70 grams per day. You might also try combining this with intermittent fasting, such as only eating within an 8-hour window, to maintain the benefits of ketosis without the side effect of fruity breath.

- – HEART PALPITATIONS

In the first few weeks of eating low carb, you might notice a slight increase in heart rate. This is probably more common in those who normally have low blood pressure.

It's often simply due to lack of salt and water, causing a reduction in the fluid circulating in the blood. This may then cause the heart to pump slightly faster or harder. So again, drink, drink, drink, and salt your foods!

This problem should go away within a week or two, but if you need to after that time, you can slightly increase your amount of carbs.

You might also want to consider a high-quality multivitamin containing zinc and selenium and a magnesium supplement to replace any nutrients lost during adaptation.

Caution For Those With Diabetes

People with diabetes should note that drastically reducing carbs can decrease the need for medicine taken to lower raised blood sugar, so taking the same amount of insulin as before could possible result in too-low blood sugar on a low-carb diet. Heart palpitations is a symptom of that.

Be sure to speak with your doctor about changes you might need to make, and test your sugar levels frequently when starting the diet.

Caution for Those with High Blood Pressure

Similar to diabetes medication, those with high blood pressure might notice that their dose becomes too strong after starting a low-carb diet, as it can improve blood pressure. Heart palpitations can also be a sign of this. Speak with your doctor about the changes and be sure to check your blood pressure at home too.

Reduced Physical Performance

You'll likely notice a large change in physical performance when first starting a low-carb way of eating, which is often caused by dehydration, lack of salt, and your body adjusting to burning fat for fuel.

It can take weeks and sometimes months for the body to adapt to the change from burning glucose for energy to using primarily fat. This part is mostly just a waiting game, but exercising while in transition might also help your body adapt faster.

Athletes are starting to experiment more with the long-term physical performance benefits of a low-carb diet, mostly those who do endurance sports and long-distance running, because there might be real advantages in performance once the body is keto- adapted. You can read more about the ketogenic diet for physical performance here.

SIDE EFFECTS OF USING A KETOGENIC DIET FOR WEIGHT LOSS

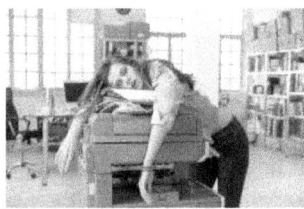

Keto Flu

This is one thing that anyone starting a ketogenic diet should brace up for. It is a condition in which you experience some of the different side effects that come along with using a ketogenic diet.

Keto flu is often characterized by light-headedness or brain fogginess, headaches, nausea, stomachaches, and muscle soreness. You may also experience heightened feelings of lethargy, irritability and trouble concentrating.

Interestingly, these are all common symptoms of the flu, hence the name. These symptoms are temporary and not everyone using a ketogenic is affected by them.

These symptoms are often caused by the sugar withdrawal occasioned by the significantly reduced carbohydrate intake. Also, an imbalance in your body electrolytes such as calcium, magnesium, potassium, and sodium can affect how your body reacts to the effect of a ketogenic diet.

Keto Breath

There are two possible reasons put forth why people on ketogenic diets experience this peculiar breath issue.

The body does not store ketones and thus they must be excreted from the body. Ketones can be excreted through the urine as acetoacetate.

They can also be excreted through the breath in form of acetone. So the more ketones you produce, the more acetone you pass out through your breath. Unfortunately, this can cause unpleasant-smelling breath when using a ketogenic diet.

On the other hand, increased protein ingestion can also cause keto breath. This is because the way the body digest fats and proteins is quite different. The digestion of proteins usually produces ammonia which the body excretes through the urine.

However, the increased consumption of proteins may result in the indigestible amounts remaining in your gut system and undergoes fermentation. This produces ammonia which is subsequently released through your breath.

Keto breath can last for about a week to just under a month. It is mostly depends on how well your body adapts to ketosis.

Micronutrient Deficiencies

This may result from the strict restrictions on carbohydrate intake. A lot of carbohydrate-rich foods are equally rich in vitamins and minerals.

The severe restriction on carbohydrate intake may therefore cause deficiencies in some essential nutrients. Therefore, we should not only be focused on the micronutrient counting in terms of fat, proteins, and carbohydrates but should also remember the vitamin and mineral micronutrient contents as well.

This is often why supplements are mostly recommended when using a ketogenic diet. Supplementation will help to augment any micronutrient imbalance that might occur when using a ketogenic diet.

AVOIDING Ketosis Side Effects

If you noticed the common theme in most of these side effects with the ketogenic diet, it involves the transition in and out of ketosis. This is one of the main reasons we have made Perfect Keto Base to eliminate any of the possible side effects as possible and ease the transition into ketosis.

The common ketosis side effects can be helped or eliminated by: drinking

more water

increasing your salt intake

and making sure you're eating enough fat

If you do still struggle with symptoms, though, a last resort would be to slightly increase the amount of carbs you're eating to alleviate symptoms. The downside to this is that it will make your low-carb diet effective less quickly, but sometimes that's necessary to continue it over the long-term.

HOW TO LOSE WEIGHT ON A KETOGENIC DIET

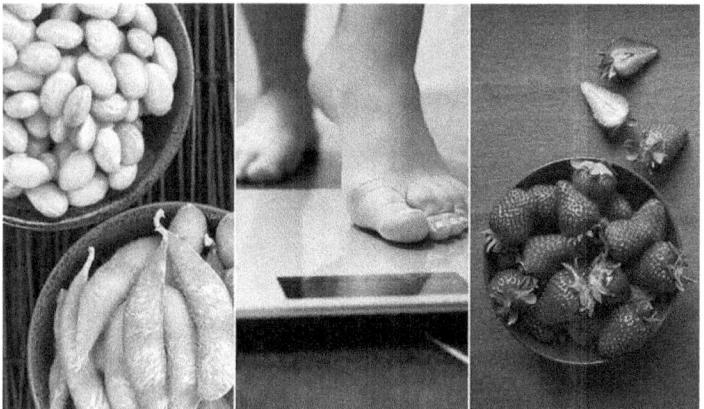

There are many ways to lose weight, and following the ketogenic diet is one of them. In fact, keto is one of the most effective ways to lose weight rapidly and keep the fat off for good.

This doesn't mean, that a high-fat, low-carb diet is ideal for everyone that is aiming for weight loss. Some people may fare better with other dietary choices that fit more snuggly into their current lifestyles.

Either way, it is possible for you to lose weight and keep it off. In this article, we will look at the research to find the most effective weight loss methods so that you can finally find something that works for you. But first, let's get a better grasp on the issue of obesity and its potential causes.

The Obesity Epidemic

More than 2 in 3 adults are considered to be overweight or have obesity in the United States. In other words, being overweight or obese is the new normal for Americans.

Unfortunately, carrying more than a few extra pounds is an epidemic throughout the world as well. Since 1975, the prevalence of obesity in the global population has tripled. Now, more than 1.9 billion adults aged 18 years and older are overweight. Of these adults, over 650 million are obese.

Each one of these people carries an increased risk of cardiovascular disease, musculoskeletal disorders (e.g., arthritis and low back pain), cancer, type 2 diabetes, and depression. What's even more frightening is that as the weight continues to increase so does the risk for this noncommunicable diseases.

And yet, despite how obvious it is that being obese is unhealthy, obesity rates are still climbing. Simply telling people to eat less and move more isn't enough — one of the primary causes of this issue runs much deeper than self-control.

The Potential Causes of The Obesity Epidemic

Just like most health issues, many different factors contribute to obesity. The factors most responsible for the obesity epidemic seem to be our genetics and the environment, and how they interact to create our eating behavior. To gain a deeper understanding of how they contribute to obesity, let's explore the organ responsible for our eating decisions the brain.

The brain was built over millions of years of genetic evolution. The evolution of the brain (and its deeply ingrained behavioral patterns) depended on its ability to adapt to an environment that shared almost nothing in common with where we spend most of our time today.

The first humans didn't have Walmart, grocery stores, and restaurants around every corner they had wild plants to forage and animals to hunt that may or may, not be there the next day. To adapt to this uncertain food environment, humans and all other animals developed a highly motivating and rewarding relationship with food.

As a result, humans and most other animals tend to eat much more than necessary in an attempt to store extra calories and other nutrients away for times when food is scarce. To put it more simply, we are wired to eat as much as possible when food is available.

More specifically, we are wired to seek out foods that contain different combinations of fat, carbs, protein, and salt. More food variety means more nutrients and better survival.

Given the choice of a fat and protein source like meat or a salt and carb rich food like potato chips, we are designed say yes to both. No matter how stuffed we are, the most primal parts of our brain will typically tell us that there is room for more if a novel food source is available. These behaviors were essential for our survival as a species. If we ate reasonably whenever food was available, then we wouldn't have enough fat or muscle to fuel us when calories were scarce.

Unfortunately, our current food environment is nothing like what the human race initially evolved to handle. Today, we are constantly bombarded with endless processed food options, food ads, and smells that trigger our desires. As a result, the oldest parts of our brain motivate us to hunt for that food, which we now have a 100% chance of getting and we don't have to exert much effort at all to get it.

We will then act out our ancestral programming by eating the most calorie dense foods (i.e., pizza, french fries, cookies, cakes, etc.) and eating much more of those foods then what our body needs to energize itself until the next meal. This results in a vicious cycle of overeating and weight gain with the subconscious intention to prepare us for famine famine that never comes.

When we consider our genetics and the current food environment together, a fascinating story reveals itself. The human species evolved from millions of years of genes that were trying to survive an environment that they didn't create. As a result, humans evolved the ability to create their own environment that allows them to fulfill their needs at any given moment with minimal effort.

The irony in all of this is that the very genes that provided us with this astounding ability to create our own food environment have not been given enough time to adapt to the abundance that the majority of the human species created for themselves.

The result? A profound mismatch between the human and its environment that causes it to eat so much and move so little that humanity accelerates its own extinction. For a more specific example, take another look at how many people are obese or overweight in the United States a country with one of the most convenient food environments.

The solution? One way of approaching this issue is through dieting. To adapt to such an abundant food environment, you need to give your brain new food rules to follow (e.g, a diet). Your brain needs you to tell it what to eat and what not to eat to meet your health goals. One of the best ways to do this is by finding a diet with simple rules that you can follow for the rest of your life.

The Best Diet For Weight Loss

Health is so complex that there is no "best diet for weight loss." Every person requires unique dietary and lifestyle changes so that they can lose weight and keep it off for the rest of their life.

What we do know for certain is that calories matter. (The human body cannot escape the laws of thermodynamics.) If you eat more than your body needs to maintain itself, then you will gain weight. Conversely, if you eat less than your body needs, then you will lose weight. It's a simple concept, but it comes with a ton of nuances.

Your daily caloric needs are not set in stone they vary slightly from day to day. Because of the unpredictable nature of our calorie requirements, many scientists have posited that they don't matter as much as other things like hormones.

The carbohydrate-insulin hypothesis, for example, proposes that the primary cause of the obesity epidemic is insulin stimulating foods like sugar and starches. The logic behind this hypothesis is based on one of the many actions of insulin.

When carbs are consumed, insulin is released by the pancreas. Once insulin interacts with fat cells, it prevents fat from being burned as fuel and triggers fat storage.

Because of this phenomenon, the supporters of the carbohydrate-insulin hypothesis tend to believe that all you need to do to lose fat is restrict carbs. However, this is a reductionistic view of obesity that doesn't account for the complex nature of the human body.

The truth is that there are multiple mechanisms for fat storage in the body that depend on calorie intake, not insulin. Insulin has also been shown to play a role in regulating our metabolic rate, which increases our caloric output to a minimal degree.

To sum up what we learned in this section, here's a helpful way to think of weight loss: Calorie intake makes the biggest impact on whether you gain or lose weight.

Other factors like exercise and insulin also matter, but to a much smaller degree.

The current literature argues between calories and carbohydrates. Below, we discuss it further.

Calories or Carbs?

Instead of focusing on switching out carbs for fat or vice versa, we should focus on sticking to a diet that naturally decreases our calorie intake.

How can we naturally decrease our calorie intake? The two most effective ways are:

Eating a diet that consists of protein-dense and fiber-rich foods because of how satiating they are.

Eliminating all calorically-dense processed foods from your diet because of how easy it is to binge on them.

One of the diets that implement this principles is the low-carb ketogenic diet. It primarily consists of highly-satiating foods like meat and low-carb vegetables while cutting out all carb-ridden, highly-palatable foods. By eating in this way, most people experience tremendous amounts of fat loss not because it lowers insulin levels, but because keto dieters tend to eat significantly fewer calories than high-carb dieters without realizing it.

Low-fat or Keto?

The meta-analysis provide us with very convincing data, but we must also consider the fact that the data came from studies where all the food was provided by the scientists. Although this is a great way to assess the difference between low-carb and high-carb diet, this does not simulate the real-world effectiveness of each diet. For this reason, we must investigate data from less strict studies. In other words, we need to look at what happened when subjects were told to follow a specific diet on their own.

They specifically looked at trials that compared a ketogenic diet that consisted of no more than 50 grams of carbs per day with a conventional, low-fat diet with less than 30% of calories from fat.

When examining the results, the researchers found that the participants in the ketogenic diet groups lost an average of 2 more pounds than the low-fat diet groups. The researchers also noted greater improvements in triglycerides, blood pressure, and HDL cholesterol in the ketogenic diet groups.

As a result, the researchers concluded that the ketogenic diet "may be an alternative tool against obesity."

These findings fall in line with another meta-analysis on 13 randomized controlled trials that compared low-fat and low-carbohydrate diets. The researchers found that, after six months, subjects who consumed less than 60 grams of carbohydrates per day had an average weight loss that was 8.8 pounds greater than the subjects on low-fat diets. At one year, the difference had fallen to 2.3 lb (which is consistent with what was found in the meta-analysis conducted by the Brazilian researchers).

As a result, the researchers concluded that "low-carbohydrate/high-protein diets are more effective at 6 months and are as effective, if not more, as low-fat diets in reducing weight and cardiovascular disease risk up to 1 year."

These two meta-analyses (and the other research you'll find in this article on keto & weight loss) provide us with a look at the real world significance of low-fat and low-carb diets. When you put people on a low-carb ketogenic type diet, they tend to lose more weight than people who are on a low-fat diet. The ketogenic diet also provides us with clear rules to follow, which makes it is easier for us to keep ourselves from overeating.

To put it another way, the ketogenic diet is one of the best ways to "hack" our brain and food environment so that we naturally eat fewer calories and lose weight. What is even more interesting is that this isn't the only reason why many people find weight loss success with keto.

Ketosis for Weight Loss

When carbohydrates are restricted for a couple of days, the body will start to produce ketones. This alternative fuel source comes with many benefits for the brain and nervous system, while it simultaneously promotes weight loss.

Once the body enters ketosis and starts to burn ketones for fuel, most ketogenic dieters will experience increased energy levels and decreased appetite. This leads to the consumption of fewer calories, resulting in more weight loss.

Another reason why ketosis and weight loss are linked is that ketones have a mild diuretic effect. This is important to know because many people will mistake their rapid weight loss on keto as if it is all coming from fat. In reality, the rapid weight loss that occurs in the first week of the ketogenic diet is mostly due to water loss.

Rapid Weight Loss on the Ketogenic Diet

Typically, during the first week of the keto diet, people see a very quick drop in weight — anywhere from 2 to 10 pounds. This is unrivaled by any other diet, but it is also not all coming from fat.

In fact, most of this weight loss is the result of the body shedding the extra water weight it was holding on to as a consequence of carbohydrate consumption. This can cause flu- like symptoms, which is why it is essential to drink plenty of water and follow the suggestions that you'll find in our guide to the keto flu.

After a week or two of keto dieting, weight loss will happen at a slower and more steady pace. This is also the period of time when the body becomes keto-adapted as it switches from burning carbs to burning fat.

How Fast Will You Lose Weight with Keto?

Once you've made it through the first week of keto and you are in ketosis, fat will steadily fall off your body (as long as you are in a calorie deficit). The average weight loss at this point is around 1-2 pounds per week the majority of it coming from fat.

As you get closer to your goal weight and your overall body weight decreases, weight loss will slow down. This happens because as your weight decreases so will your daily caloric needs. For this reason, you may want to recalculate your calorie needs every month or so.

Keep in mind that weight loss may, not be consistent either. You might have some weeks where it seems you haven't lost anything then you'll weigh yourself a week or two later and be down 3-4 pounds.

How Fast Will You Lose Weight with Keto?

What is behind the seemingly unpredictable and unique nature of your weight loss rate? Here are some of the critical factors that determine how fast the pounds will come off:

Your calorie deficit. The one factor that leads to the most significant and consistent weight loss is a calorie deficit. In other words, when we consume fewer calories than we need to maintain our weight, we will lose weight. This means that your weight loss rate will usually increase as your total calorie consumption decreases. However, there are limits to how far you should take you should take your deficit. The human body is designed to prevent massive amounts of weight loss during times of starvation via mechanisms that make long-term fat loss much harder to achieve and maintain. Because of this, it is never a good idea to starve yourself for extended periods of time. Research indicates that calorie deficits above 30% are enough to stimulate some of these counterproductive mechanisms for long-term fat loss.

Your current health status. Your overall health plays a major role in how fast you will lose weight and adapt to a lower carb diet. If you have any hormonal or metabolic issues, weight loss might be slower or a bit more challenging than expected. Insulin resistance, excess visceral fat, and thyroid issues, for example, can all have a significant impact on your weight loss rate.

Your body composition. Do you have a lot of fat to lose? How much muscle do you have? The people who have the most to lose will tend to shred the fat at a much faster rate than those who have a few extra pounds to burn off. This phenomenon is mostly explained by the fact that obese individuals can easily maintain a much larger calorie deficit, which will result in faster weight loss. Muscle mass also plays a vital role in weight loss because it helps keep your metabolic rate from dropping significantly as you lose weight. This can help stabilize your weight loss rate and may even prevent a dreaded weight loss plateau.

Your daily habits. Your daily habits will make or break your weight loss efforts. Consistency is the key to keto success. Are you eating clean keto foods or high-fat junk foods with low-quality ingredients? Are you watching out for hidden carbs? Are you exercising? Eating the right foods in the right amounts for your goals and adding more physical activity to your daily life is the most important pieces of a smooth and successful body transformation.

When we take a step back and look at the bigger picture of our fat loss rate, predictable patterns began to emerge. For example, the people who typically see the slowest weight loss are those who are sedentary and overweight with poor metabolic health and eating habits that don't exercise or keep track of their carb and/or calorie consumption.

Conversely, those who start with more muscle and decent metabolic health that are disciplined enough to stick to their diet plan, maintain a calorie deficit, and increase their physical activity levels will typically lose weight more quickly and get the results they want.

In general, everyone's health and lifestyle is different, which means the weight loss rate for each person is going to be different too. We do, however, share one thing in common: each one of us can optimize our body composition with our diets.

How Much Weight Loss Will You Get from Following the Keto Diet?

With a well-formulated keto diet, you can technically drop as much fat as you want.

Yes, you read that correctly – you have the potential to sculpt your body into incredible shape with keto. However, most of us will not reach our body composition goals by simple restricting carbs and being in ketosis.

From a dietary perspective, getting the results that you desire will take discipline, consistency, and a well-formulated, healthy dietary approach. The discipline and consistency are up to you; our job is to provide you with the information that will help you reach your goals with the keto diet.

To help you get started on your weight loss journey, we put together a list of the four fundamental principles that will help you formulate a healthy keto diet for your needs:

Eat the right amount of calories and protein to meet your goals. You can use our keto calculator and calorie tracking guide to help you with this.

Get most of your calories from micronutrient dense foods. For more detailed information on what to eat, check out our guide to micronutrients and our keto food list.

Make sure your diet is improving your overall health and wellbeing subjectively and objectively.

Implement lifestyle adjustments to make your diet into a long-term lifestyle that you can follow indefinitely.

You will know that you are following a well-formulated and healthy keto diet for you if these four variables are trending in the right direction:

Your mood, energy levels, and sense of well-being Your

body composition

Relevant biomarkers (e.g., blood pressure, cholesterol, triglyceride, and blood sugar levels)

Your ketone levels

For more information on how to create a keto diet that is healthy and effective for you, we recommend checking out our recent article on the topic.

However, even if you follow every suggestion and strategy flawlessly, you may end up stalling at the same weight for a few weeks. In this case, you may need to make some minor adjustments to your diet to get back on track.

How to Break Through Plateaus and Boost Weight Loss on the Ketogenic Diet

Plateaus are an inevitable part of every diet. Eventually, you will get to a point where you are eating what your body needs to maintain its weight. This can happen months to years after you start the keto diet.

When you encounter the dreaded plateau, don't give up simply follow some of these suggestions:

Track your calories. If you are not already doing so, track your calories using an app like Cronometer. This simple habit will take your results to the next level because you'll have an objective way of knowing if you are eating the right amount of carbs, fat, protein, and calories every day.

Recalculate your macronutrient targets. When you hit a plateau or simply want to boost your fat loss, plug your updated information into the keto calculator. This will allow you to maintain a calorie deficit even after your calorie needs have dropped.

Experiment with fat fasting. If you are still struggling, try implementing a technique called the fat fast. It normally consists of a three-day window of low caloric intake and high amounts of fat to kickstart fat burning and increase fat loss. If you're interested, I went into more detail on fat fasting in another post.

Eat less often. It's much easier to eat fewer calories and maintain higher levels of ketosis when you eat less meals. Instead of snacking throughout the day, try getting all of your calories from 2-3 meals every day. You can also try intermittent fasting by restricting all your meals to an 8-hour eating window. This will allow your blood sugar and insulin to drop down to baseline levels so that your body can go into its fasting state and burn body fat for fuel.

Stick to the ketogenic diet (no cheating). Going from keto to high-carb will cause you to gain weight rapidly. Even just one cheat day can cause you to gain 4 to 6 pounds of water weight. If you have a sugar craving, indulge in a keto-friendly dessert instead of a sugar-filled snack.

Don't eat foods that you are sensitive to. If your body struggles with dairy, gluten, or other foods in any way, then consider eliminating it from your diet. Food sensitivities can slow progress and impair health.

Check for hidden carb sources. You may be eating more carbs than you think. Make sure you aren't getting too many carbs from sneaky sources like vegetables, peanut butter, processed meats, and over-the-counter medications.

Decrease your stress levels. The most common ways that people stress their bodies on a diet is by eating too little and exercising too much. Studies have found that exercising for more than an hour a day can drop our metabolic rate by 15%, and maintaining a caloric deficit of 25% can decrease our metabolic rate by 6%. In other words, don't overdo it you will slow your metabolism down and cause your own weight loss plateau.

Eat the right amount of protein. Too much protein can increase insulin levels and decrease ketone levels, while not consuming enough protein can cause you to burn muscle rather than fat. If you exercise, protein levels should be hovering around 0.8g – 1.0g protein per lean pound of body mass a day. This helps with muscle mass retention and growth. However, if you are not exercising – your protein intake doesn't need to be as high. A protein intake of 0.6g – 0.8g of protein per lean pound of body mass is going to be fine for sedentary individuals.

Lift weights. By lifting weights, you will build muscle mass and modestly increase your metabolic rate and fat loss. One of the best ways to increase muscle mass is by doing bodybuilding type workouts. For an overview of how to gain muscle on keto, check out our guide to keto bodybuilding.

Take calorie deficit breaks. If nothing else seems to work, then try taking intermittent diet breaks every two weeks or so. Recent research found that obese men who took 2 week breaks from being in a caloric deficit lost more fat than the men who maintained a calorie deficit. This means that keto dieters may benefit from taking intermittent calorie deficit breaks as well. To implement a diet break, simply follow the ketogenic diet for two weeks while you maintain a calorie deficit. After that two weeks, calculate what you need to eat to maintain your bodyweight, aim to eat that many calories, and repeat recalculating your calorie deficit after each calorie maintenance phase. Researchers hypothesize that this method of dieting helps keep your metabolism from slowing down, allowing you to burn more calories while you are in a calorie deficit.

Looking for more specific info on how to bust through weight loss plateaus on the ketogenic diet? Follow this link to learn more.

However, there is one caveat when it comes to weight loss. In response to a calorie deficit, the body will typically burn some of its muscle mass for fuel by using a process called gluconeogenesis. As a result, many people will lose muscle along with the fat when they diet. Luckily, there is a way to preserve muscle mass, even in the midst of extreme caloric deficits.

How To Avoid Muscle Loss On Keto

The most important macronutrient for preserving and building lean muscle is protein. Carbs help preserve muscle mass to some extent, but protein is — without a doubt — the most important macronutrient that you must eat enough if you don't want to lose muscle.

Protein consumption is especially crucial on the ketogenic diet. Without dietary carbs to provoke an anabolic (muscle building) response, you will tend to lose muscle more rapidly without adequate protein intake on keto.

With that being said, research has also found that ketones have a muscle preserving effect. Because of this, it is reasonable to suggest that you should eat just enough protein to maintain muscle mass without eating so much protein that you decrease your ketone levels.

How To Avoid Muscle Loss On Keto

Here is the protein intake that we recommend for keto dieters:

If you exercise, protein levels should be hovering around 0.8g – 1.0g protein per lean pound of body mass a day.

If you are sedentary, then your protein intake should be between 0.6g – 0.8g per lean pound of body mass.

The higher the caloric deficit, the closer your protein intake should be to the higher end of the range.

Keep in mind, however, that consuming too much protein at any given meal can decrease your levels of ketosis. To mitigate this effect, you can divide your protein intake into equal amounts throughout your meals. If you workout, then consider consuming more protein after and/or before your workouts because this protein is less likely to spike insulin levels and reduce ketone levels.

However, even if you follow all the recommendations in this article, you still won't know for certain if you are actually losing fat. To get a more accurate measure of your fat loss, it is essential to estimate and track your body fat percentage.

How to Track Your Fat Loss on the Ketogenic Diet

There are many methods you can use to evaluate your fat loss, but the two simplest ways are by visually estimating your body fat percentage and by plugging your waist circumference, height, and weight into a body fat calculator.

On the other hand, if you'd like to use a body fat calculator, here's what you do: Wrap the

tape measure around your waist at the level of your belly button.

Exhale all your air and secure the tape without stretching it.

Read the measurement, write it down, and calculate your percentage of body fat by plugging it into this body fat calculator.

Remeasure every 2 to 4 weeks to track your progress.

How to Track Your Fat Loss on the Ketogenic Diet

Although this isn't particularly accurate, it will provide you with a reasonable estimate of your body fat % that you can track while you are dieting. You can also look at your body fat % estimate along with your weight and waist circumference to determine if the weight you lost is fat or water.

Waist circumference, for example, tends to decrease as fat mass decreases, providing you with an indicator that you lost fat. If your goal is to gain muscle mass and lose fat, then the numbers on the scale should either increase or stay the same as the numbers on the measuring tape and your body fat % calculation decrease.

Losing Weight on Keto

The bulk of research suggests that the ketogenic diet is more effective than conventional diets in helping you lose weight and shed body fat. One of the reasons why the ketogenic diet provides such reliable weight loss results is because it consists primarily of highly- satiating whole foods like meat, high-fat dairy, and low-carb vegetables while removing all carb-rich, sugar-laden processed foods from the diet. By eating in this way, you will feel full while eating fewer calories and losing weight.

The most important part of the ketogenic diet is consistency. Approach this diet (or any other diet that you try) with the mindset that you will make it into a long-term sustainable lifestyle. When you hit a plateau, don't give up we all hit plateaus eventually. Take it as an opportunity to recalculate your calorie needs, adjust your goals, and implement new strategies.

To maximize your fat loss on keto even further, follow these suggestions: Track your macronutrient consumption

Aim to reduce your waist circumference and body fat % Eat the right amount of protein

Reduce your stress levels Lift weights

Supplement your diet with MCTs and CLA

USES OF THE KETOGENIC DIET

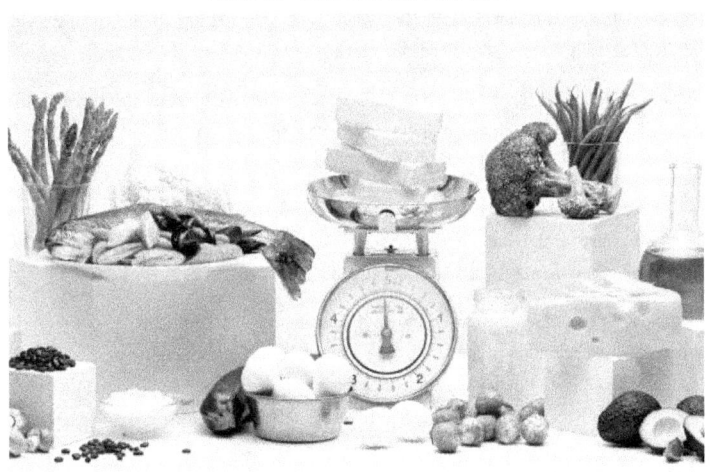

When using a ketogenic diet, your body becomes more of a fat-burner than a carbohydrate-dependent machine. Several researches have linked the consumption of increased amounts of carbohydrates to development of several disorders such as diabetes and insulin resistance.

By nature, carbohydrates are easily absorbable and therefore can be also be easily stored by the body. Digestion of carbohydrates starts right from the moment you put them into your mouth.

As soon as you begin chewing them, amylase (the enzymes that digest carbohydrate) in your saliva is already at work acting on the carbohydrate-containing food.

In the stomach, carbohydrates are further broken down. When they get into the small intestines, they are then absorbed into the bloodstream. On getting to the bloodstream, carbohydrates generally increase the blood sugar level.

This increase in blood sugar level stimulates the immediate release of insulin into the bloodstream. The higher the increase in blood sugar levels, the more the amount of insulin that is release.

Insulin is a hormone that causes excess sugar in the bloodstream to be removed in order to lower the blood sugar level. Insulin takes the sugar and carbohydrate that you eat and stores them either as glycogen in muscle tissues or as fat in adipose tissue for future use as energy.

However, the body can develop what is known as insulin resistance when it is continuously exposed to such high amounts of glucose in the bloodstream. This scenario can easily cause obesity as the body tends to quickly store any excess amount of glucose. Health conditions such as diabetes and cardiovascular disease can also result from this condition.

Keto diets are low in carbohydrate and high in fat and have been associated with reducing and improving several health conditions.

One of the foremost things a ketogenic diet does is to stabilize your insulin levels and also restore leptin signalling. Reduced amounts of insulin in the bloodstream allow you to feel fuller for a longer period of time and also to have fewer cravings.

Medical Benefits of Ketogenic Diets

The application and implementation of the ketogenic diet has expanded considerably. Keto diets are often indicated as part of the treatment plan in a number of medical conditions.

Epilepsy

This is basically the main reason for the development of the ketogenic diet. For some reason, the rate of epileptic seizures reduces when patients are placed on a keto diet.

Pediatric epileptic cases are the most responsive to the keto diet. There are children who have experience seizure elimination after a few years of using a keto diet.

Children with epilepsy is generally expected to fast for a few days before starting the ketogenic diet as part of their treatment.

Cancer

Research suggests that the therapeutic efficacy of the ketogenic diets against tumor growth can be enhanced when combined with certain drugs and procedures under a "press-pulse" paradigm.

It is also promising to note that ketogenic diets drive the cancer cell into remission. This means that keto diets "starves cancer" to reduce the symptoms.

Alzheimer Disease

There are several indications that the memory functions of patients with Alzheimer's disease improve after making use of a ketogenic diet.

Ketones are a great source of alternative energy for the brain especially when it has become resistant to insulin. Ketones also provide substrates (cholesterol) that help to repair damaged neurons and membranes. These all help to improve memory and cognition in Alzheimer patients.

Diabetes

It is generally agreed that carbohydrates are the main culprit in diabetes. Therefore, by reducing the amount of ingested carbohydrate by using a ketogenic diet, there are increased chances for improved blood sugar control.

Also, combining a keto diet with other diabetes treatment plans can significantly improve their overall effectiveness.

Gluten Allergy

Many individuals with gluten allergy are undiagnosed with this condition. However, following a ketogenic diet showed improvement in related symptoms like digestive discomforts and bloating.

Most carbohydrate-rich foods are high in gluten. Thus, by using a keto diet, a lot of the gluten consumption is reduced to a minimum due to the elimination of a large variety of carbohydrates.

Weight Loss

This is arguably the most common "intentional" use of the ketogenic diet today. It has found a niche for itself in the mainstream dieting trend. Keto diets have become part of many dieting regimen due to its well acknowledged side effect of aiding weight loss.

Though initially maligned by many, the growing number of favorable weight loss results has helped the ketogenic to better embraced as a major weight loss program.

Besides the above medical benefits, ketogenic diets also provide some general health benefits which include the following.

Improved Insulin Sensitivity

This is obviously the first aim of a ketogenic diet. It helps to stabilize your insulin levels thereby improving fat burning.

Muscle Preservation

Since protein is oxidized, it helps to preserve lean muscle. Losing lean muscle mass causes an individual's metabolism to slow down as muscles are generally very metabolic. Using a keto diet actually helps to preserve your muscles while your body burns fat.

Controlled pH and respiratory function

A ketoc diet helps to decrease lactate thereby improving both pH and respiratory function. A state of ketosis therefore helps to keep your blood pH at a healthy level.

Improved Immune System

Using a ketogenic diet helps to fight off aging antioxidants while also reducing inflammation of the gut thereby making your immune system stronger.

Reduced Cholesterol Levels

Consuming fewer carbohydrates while you are on the keto diet will help to reduce blood cholesterol levels. This is due to the increased state of lipolysis. This leads to a reduction in LDL cholesterol levels and an increase in HDL cholesterol levels.

Reduced Appetite and Cravings

Adopting a ketogenic diet helps you to reduce both your appetite and cravings for calorie rich foods. As you begin eating healthy, satisfying, and beneficial high-fat foods, your hunger feelings will naturally start decreasing.

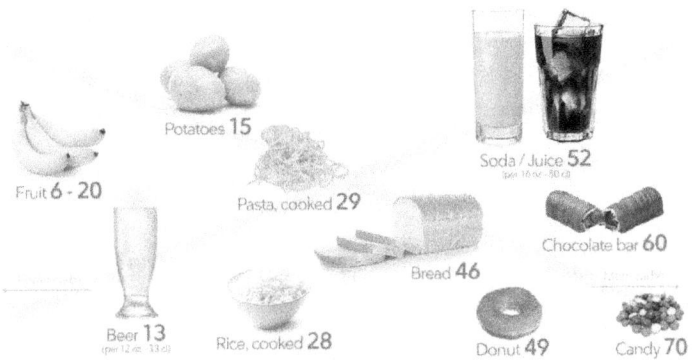

Potatoes 15

Soda / Juice 52
per 16 oz - 50 cl

Fruit 6 - 20

Pasta, cooked 29

Chocolate bar 60

Bread 46

Beer 13
per 12 oz - 33 cl

Rice, cooked 28

Donut 49

Candy 70

A ketogenic diet is basically a diet which converts your body from burning sugar to burning fat. Around 99% of the wold's population have a diet which cause their body to burn sugar. As a result, carbohydrates are their primary fuel source used after digesting carbs. This process makes people gain weight, however a diet of fat and ketones will cause weight loss. As you ask what can you eat on a ketogenic diet, first of all eat up to 30 to 50 grams of carbs per day. Next, let us discover more about what you can have on your plate and how the ketogenic diet affects your health.

The Importance Of Sugar Precaution On The Ketogenic Diet

Keto shifts your body from a sugar burner to a fat burner by eliminating the dietary sugar derived from carbohydrates. The first obvious reduction you should make from your current diet is sugar and sugary foods. Although sugar is a definite target for deletion, the ketogenic diet focuses upon the limitation of carbohydrates. We need to watch out for sugar in a number of different types of foods and nutrients. Even a white potato which is carb-heavy may not taste sweet to your tongue like sugar. But once it hits your bloodstream after digestion, those carbs add the simple sugar known as glucose to your body. The truth is, our body can only store so much glucose before it dumps it elsewhere in our system. Excess glucose becomes what is known as the fat which accumulates in our stomach region, love handles, etc.

Protein And It's Place In Keto

One source of carbohydrates which some people overlook in their diet is protein. Overconsumption of protein according to the tolerance level of your body will result in weight gain. Because our body converts excess protein into sugar, we must moderate the amount of protein we eat. Moderation of our protein intake is part of how to eat ketogenic and lose weight. First of all, identify your own tolerance of daily protein and use as a guide to maintain an optimal intake of the nutrient. Second, choose your protein from foods such as organic cage-free eggs and grass-fed meats. Finally, create meals in variety that are delicious and maintain your interest in the diet. For instance, a 5 ounce steak and a few eggs can provide an ideal amount of daily protein for some people.

Caloric Intake On The Ketogenic Diet

Calories are another important consideration for what can you eat on a ketogenic diet. Energy derived from the calories in the food we consume help our body to remain functional. Hence, we must eat enough calories in order to meet our daily nutritional requirements. Counting calories is a burden for many people who are on other diets. But as a ketogenic dieter, you don't have to worry nearly as much about calorie counting. Most people on a low-carb diet remain satisfied by eating a daily amount of 1500-1700 kcals in calories.

Fats, The Good & The Bad

Fat is not bad, in fact many good healthy fats exist in whole foods such as nuts, seeds and olive oil. Healthy fats are an integral part of the ketogenic diet and are available as spreads, snacks and toppings. Misconceptions in regards to eating fat are that a high amount of it is unhealthy and causes weight gain. While both statements are in a sense true, the fat which we consume is not the direct cause of the fat which appears on our body. Rather, the sugar from each nutrient we consume is what eventually becomes the fat on our body.

Balance Your Nutrients Wisely

Digestion causes the sugars we eat to absorb into the bloodstream and the excess amount transfer into our fat cells. High carbohydrate and high protein eating will result in excess body fat, because there is sugar content in these nutrients. So excessive eating of any nutrient is unhealthy and causes weight gain. But a healthy diet consists of a balance of protein, carbohydrates and fats according to the tolerance levels of your body.

Just about everyone can accomplish a ketogenic diet with enough persistence and effort. In addition, we can moderate a number of bodily conditions naturally with keto. Insulin resistance, elevated blood sugar, inflammation, obesity, type-2 diabetes are some health conditions that keto can help to stabilize. Each of these unhealthy conditions will reduce and normalize for the victim who follows a healthy ketogenic diet. Low-carb, high-fat and moderate protein whole foods provide the life-changing health benefits of this diet.

WHAT ARE THE SIGNS OF KETOSIS

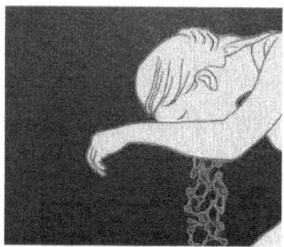

Ketosis is a metabolic process that occurs when the body begins to burn fat for energy because it does not have enough carbohydrates to burn. During this process, the liver produces chemicals called ketones.

The ketogenic, or keto, diet aims to induce ketosis in order to burn more fat. Proponents of the diet claim that it boosts weight loss and improves overall health.

Despite these guidelines, some people following the diet may not know when they are in ketosis.

we list 10 signs and symptoms that may help a person determine whether the ketogenic diet is working for them.

1 Increased ketones

A blood sample can indicate ketone levels.

Having ketones in the blood is probably the most definitive sign that someone is in ketosis. Doctors may also use urine and breath tests to check for ketone levels, but these are less reliable than blood samples.

A special home testing kit allows people to measure their own blood ketone levels. Or, a doctor may take a blood sample and send it away for testing. When a person is in nutritional ketosis, they will have blood ketone levels of 0.5–3 millimoles per liter.

Alternatively, people can use a breath analyzer to test for ketones in their breath, or they may use indicator strips to check their urinary levels.

2 Weight loss

Some research suggests that this type of very-low-carbohydrate diet is effective for weight loss. Therefore, people should expect to lose some weight when in ketosis.

The results of 2013 meta-analysis that examined the findings from several randomized controlled trials suggest that people following a ketogenic diet may lose more weight in the long-term than people following a low-fat diet.

People on a ketogenic diet may notice weight loss in the first few days, but this is typically just a reduction in water weight. True fat loss may not occur for several weeks.

3 Thirst

Ketosis may cause some people to feel thirstier than usual, which may occur as a side effect of water loss. However, high levels of ketones in the body can also lead to dehydration and an electrolyte imbalance. Both of these reactions can cause complications.

Research into ketogenic diets for sports performance lists dehydration as a side effect of ketosis. Athletes may also have a higher risk of kidney stones, which is a complication of dehydration.

To avoid dehydration, drink plenty of water and other liquids. See a doctor if symptoms of dehydration, such as extreme thirst or dark-colored urine, occur.

4 Muscle cramps and spasms

Dehydration and electrolyte imbalances can cause muscle cramps. Electrolytes are substances that carry electrical signals between the body's cells. Imbalances in these substances lead to disrupted electrical messages that may cause muscle contractions and spasms.

People following the ketogenic diet should ensure that they are getting enough electrolytes from the food they eat to avoid muscle pains and other symptoms of an imbalance.

Electrolytes include calcium, magnesium, potassium, and sodium. A person can get these from eating a balanced diet. However, if symptoms persist, a doctor may recommend supplements or other dietary changes.

5 Headaches

Ketosis headaches can last from 1 to 7 days, or longer.

Headaches can be a common side effect of switching to a ketogenic diet. They may occur as a result of consuming fewer carbohydrates, especially sugar. Dehydration and electrolyte imbalances can also cause headaches.

Ketosis headaches typically last from 1 day to 1 week, although some people may experience pain for longer. See a doctor if headaches persist.

6 Fatigue and weakness

In the initial stages of a ketosis diet, people may feel more tired and weaker than usual. This fatigue occurs as the body switches from burning carbohydrates to burning fat for energy. Carbohydrates provide a quicker burst of energy to the body.

A small 2017 study involving athletes found tiredness to be a common side effect of the ketosis diet. Participants typically observed this during the first few weeks.

After several weeks on the diet, people should notice an increase in their energy levels. If not, they should seek medical attention, as fatigue is also a symptom of dehydration and nutrient deficiencies.

7 Stomach complaints

Making any dietary changes can raise the risk of stomach upset and other digestive complaints. This may also occur when a person switches to the ketogenic diet.

To reduce the risk of experiencing stomach complaints, drink plenty of water and other fluids. Eat non-starchy vegetables and other fiber-rich foods to alleviate constipation, and consider taking a probiotic supplement to encourage a healthy gut.

8 Changes in sleep

Following a ketogenic diet may disrupt a person's sleeping habits. Initially, they may experience difficulty falling asleep or nighttime waking. These symptoms typically go away within a few weeks.

9 Bad breath

A common side effect of ketosis is bad breath.

Bad breath is among the most common side effects of ketosis. This is because ketones leave the body through the breath as well as the urine. People on the diet, or those around them, may notice that the breath smells sweet or fruity.

A ketone called acetone is usually responsible for the odor, but other ketones, such as benzophenone and acetophenone, may also contribute to bad breath.

There is no way to reduce ketosis breath, but it may improve with time. Some people use sugar-free gum or brush their teeth several times per day to mask the smell.

10 Better focus and concentration

Initially, the ketogenic diet may cause headaches and concentration difficulties. However, these symptoms should fade over time. People following a long-term ketogenic diet often report better clarity and focus, and some research supports this.

According to the results of a 2018 systematic review, people with epilepsy who follow the ketogenic diet report better alertness and attention. Also, these people showed greater alertness in some cognitive tests.

A KETOGENIC DIET FOR PHYSICAL PERFORMANCE

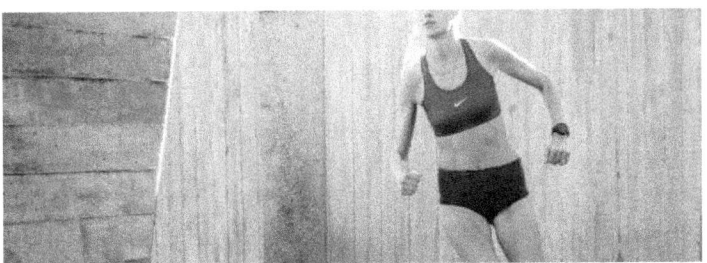

Should those who are physically active continue eating low-carb? It's a fair question for those wanting to follow a ketogenic diet for better health, and that's why we'll be exploring the main areas of ketosis for physical performance.

The ketogenic diet and ketosis have been used traditionally by physicians and other professionals for a few different medical reasons, including improving the health of those with diabetes and treating neurological disorders like epilepsy.

But now, we've begun to explore other factors where the ketogenic diet can have a positive effect, including mental focus, weight loss, and in this article, ketosis for physical performance.

The Ketogenic Diet for Exercise

While the emphasis for exercise is usually on high carbohydrate intake, the ketogenic diet takes a low-carb approach to energy. Those on a ketogenic diet generally stay within a range of 30-50 grams of carbs per day, and a large amount of food in the diet comes from fat.

The ketogenic diet involves a dietary breakdown of: Low

carbohydrate intake

Moderate protein intake High

fat intake

The low intake of carbs is meant to put the dieter into ketosis, where the body creates ketones from fat stores to use as the main energy source, instead of carbs, for the body and even partly for the brain. Molecules known as ketones are produced during the process.

This means that someone exercising while eating a ketogenic diet is going to be using primarily fat as fuel for their physical activity.

Misconceptions About Ketosis For Physical Performance

A long-held belief among the nutrition and medical community is that carbohydrates must make up a high portion of your diet in order to maintain physical performance at an ideal level. This belief mostly stems from studies in the last 100 years looking at muscle glycogen and its link to high intensity exercise.

However, there are few reasons to question this thought process:

We've observed cultures that didn't eat in line with the carb-heavy philosophy, such as the Inuit people in the Canadian and Alaskan Arctic regions. Before their diets changed a lot, scientists were able to observe their traditional diet and see that it contained virtually no known carbohydrates, yet they were able to function normally physically.

Demographic evidence of past European cultures has shown them living as primarily hunters without any noted physical impediments.

While diets with more carbohydrates may prove better for higher-intensity, short-term forms of exercise, the limitations of the ketogenic diet for physical performance have been over exaggerated. In fact, ketosis can have a healthy role in relation physical activity for most individuals.

Let's take a look at the differences associated with using ketones for fuel versus using carbs for fuel.

Fat Adaptation In Ketosis

With a ketogenic or other low carb diet, the body experiences fat adaptation, or keto- adaption, where it becomes more efficient at burning fat and ketones for fuel. This adaptation can be strong and have a great impact on the fat burning process during exercise.

During a recent study, ultra-endurance athletes who were on a ketogenic diet for an average of 20 months were shown to burn up to 2.3 times more fat than the high-carb group during a three-hour run. The study also found that muscle glycogen use and repletion during and after the exercise was similar between the low-carb and high-carb groups. This is a significant demonstration of the power of keto-adaptation for exercise.

Endurance Exercise And Ketosis

As we've established, fat can be used for energy when carbs aren't available for use. While carbs do provide more fuel for the body to perform at higher intensities, fat is what provides more energy during exercise at lower intensities.

However, this might be open to question as well. In one study, researchers recorded athletes following a ketogenic diet had burned mostly fat during exercise at up to 70% of their max intensity, while the high-carb athletes burned fat at 55%. This again demonstrates the increased effectiveness of ketosis for fuel during exercise when a person's body has adapted to burning primarily fat for energy.

With this in mind, it's still important to recognize that some elite athletes may require energy more quickly than the rate at which they can get it from fat, and more research is needed on the subject to know the details for sure.

That being said, a low-carb ketogenic diet can be helpful in regards to exercise for:

Preventing tiredness when doing longer exercise

Perform low-to-moderate intensity levels of exercise through keto-adaptation Improving

health and losing more fat through regular exercise and low-carb eating Maintaining

blood glucose during exercise

Adapting the body to burning more fat, which might be able to help the body preserve glycogen in the muscles during exercise

Muscle Growth And Ketosis

We don't currently have research showing a specific benefit of ketogenic diets over higher carb diets for muscle growth during strength or high-intensity exercises. That being said, there are some studies show that in addition to using more fat as fuel, low- carb diets can also help preserve muscle glycogen for some athletes. Plus, a ketogenic diet has the advantage of teaching the body to more easily turn to fat burning for fuel.

However, that doesn't mean it's necessary to turn to a very high carb diet to see success in muscle growth and performance. In fact, a diet that is higher in protein and more moderate in carb intake might be the best for achieving ideal body composition and muscle growth for most active people and some sports athletes.

An Early Account Of Ketogenic Diet Performance

Let's take a second to travel back over a hundred years ago to one of the earliest recorded examples of a ketogenic diet for intense physical performance.

Benefits Of Ketosis For Athletes

A lower carb intake does have some potential benefits for certain types of athletes. For example:

Some research shows that the preservation of glycogen stores from a ketogenic diet can prevent endurance athletes from "hitting the wall" while performing endurance exercises.

Keto-adaptation can lead to less reliance on carbs during endurance exercise, which can help athletes during events where there is limited access to food or those who can't easily digest carbs during exercise.

A diet that promotes more fat loss is important for improve the ratio of fat to muscle, which is crucial for those looking to improve their exercise performance or meet certain weight goals for their sport, such as in wrestling, weightlifting, and boxing.

The practice of exercising while glycogen stores are low is a training technique popular for improving the function of mitochondria, enzymes, and fat usage to improve overall health and physical performance long-term.

Eating a ketogenic diet might also be a good diet practice for an athlete's off season as they maintain their health while resting.

While the jury is still out on the benefits of a ketogenic diet over a higher carb diet for all athletes, ketosis for physical performance can be helpful for those doing ultra- endurance or low-intensity exercise meant to maintain health.

WHAT IS KETO FLU

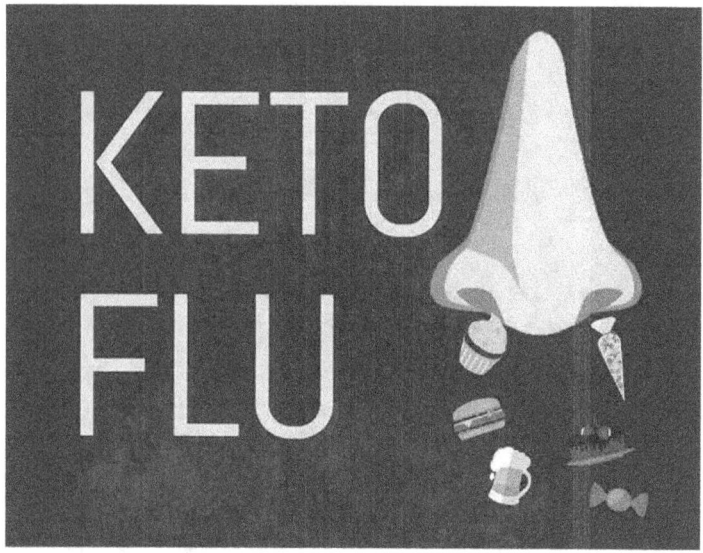

Many people have decided to try the ketogenic diet for weight loss. The most recent evidence shows that reducing your carbohydrate intake to a minimum may help you shed a few pounds, at least in the first few weeks to months. However, we don't really know whether, over the long term, achieving and maintaining ketosis is better for weight loss than other diets. Almost any intervention can cause undesirable consequences, and the ketogenic diet is no different. One of the most well-publicized complications of ketosis is something called "keto flu."

What is keto flu?

The so-called keto flu is a group of symptoms that may appear two to seven days after starting a ketogenic diet. Headache, foggy brain, fatigue, irritability, nausea, difficulty sleeping, and constipation are just some of the symptoms of this condition, which is not recognized by medicine. A search for this term yields not a single result on PubMed, the library of indexed medical research journals. On the other hand, an internet search will yield thousands of blogs and articles about keto flu.

It is tricky to describe exactly what happens after the diet change, because we are left with only our own observations and experiences. These symptoms may not even be unique to the ketogenic diet; some of my patients describe similar symptoms after they cut back on processed foods, or decide to follow an elimination or an anti-inflammatory diet.

What causes keto flu?

Well, we don't really know why some people feel so bad after this dietary change. Is it related to a detox factor? Is it due to a carb withdrawal? Is there an immunologic reaction? Or is this a result of a change in the gut microbiome? Whatever the reason is, it appears the symptoms attributed to the keto flu may happen, not to everyone but to some people, after "cleaning up" their diet.

What to do for keto flu?

If you decide for whatever reason to change your diet and feel tired and a little off, do not become exasperated and lose hope. Here are few tips:

Supercharge your cold and flu defenses!

Surprising secrets, smart strategies, and simple steps to keep your immune system at its cold-and-flu-fighting best

Get the tips to stay healthy

There is no need to go online and buy any expensive supplements. Many websites are trying to make big bucks selling products to make you feel better without any data to back up those claims.

Despite its name, this is not like the flu. You will not develop a fever and the symptoms can hardly ever make you incapacitated. If you feel very ill, consider visiting your doctor, as something else may be happening.

Make sure you drink plenty of water. Some diets can make you dehydrated.

Eat more often and make sure you have plenty of colorful vegetables. Switching from a standard American diet, rich in simple carbs, trans fats, and saturated fat, is a big change in how your cells use energy. Food is not only calories and energy, it is communication to your cells.

Do not give up if you are committed to a plan. You may feel exhausted for a few days, but at the end of a week, your energy level will most likely return to normal and you may feel even better.

If everything else fails, consider easing into the new diet more slowly, instead of "cold turkey."

Undesirable symptoms may show up in the first few days after changing what you eat. But this should not be the deciding factor when choosing what to put on your plate.

How To Get Rid Of The Keto Flu

The keto flu can make you feel miserable.

Luckily, there are ways to reduce its flu-like symptoms and help your body get through the transition period more easily.

Stay Hydrated

Drinking enough water is necessary for optimal health and can also help reduce symptoms.

A keto diet can cause you to rapidly shed water stores, increasing the risk of dehydration

This is because glycogen, the stored form of carbohydrates, binds to water in the body. When dietary carbohydrates are reduced, glycogen levels plummet and water is excreted from the body

Staying hydrated can help with symptoms like fatigue and muscle cramping

Replacing fluids is especially important when you are experiencing keto-flu-associated diarrhea, which can cause additional fluid loss

Avoid Strenuous Exercise

While exercise is important for staying healthy and keeping body weight in check, strenuous exercise should be avoided when experiencing keto-flu symptoms.

Fatigue, muscle cramps and stomach discomfort are common in the first week of following a ketogenic diet, so it may be a good idea to give your body a rest.

Activities like intense biking, running, weight lifting and strenuous workouts may have to be put on the back burner while your system adapts to new fuel sources.

While these types of exercise should be avoided if you are experiencing the keto flu, light activities like walking, yoga or leisurely biking may improve symptoms.

Replace Electrolytes

Replacing dietary electrolytes may help reduce keto-flu symptoms.

When following a ketogenic diet, levels of insulin, an important hormone that helps the body absorb glucose from the bloodstream, decrease.

When insulin levels decrease, the kidneys release excess sodium from the body

What's more, the keto diet restricts many foods that are high in potassium, including fruits, beans and starchy vegetables.

Getting adequate amounts of these important nutrients is an excellent way to power through the adaptation period of the diet.

Salting food to taste and including potassium-rich, keto-friendly foods like green leafy vegetables and avocados are an excellent way to ensure you are maintaining a healthy balance of electrolytes.

These foods are also high in magnesium, which may help reduce muscle cramps, sleep issues and headaches

Get Adequate Sleep

Fatigue and irritability are common complaints of people who are adapting to a ketogenic diet.

Lack of sleep causes levels of the stress hormone cortisol to rise in the body, which can negatively impact mood and make keto-flu symptoms worse

If you are having a difficult time falling or staying asleep, try one of the following tips:

Reduce caffeine intake: Caffeine is a stimulant that may negatively impact sleep. If you drink caffeinated beverages, only do so in the morning so your sleep is not affected

Cut out ambient light: Shut off cell phones, computers and televisions in the bedroom to create a dark environment and promote restful sleep

Take a bath: Adding Epsom salt or lavender essential oil to your bath is a relaxing way to wind down and get ready for sleep

Get up early: Waking at the same time every day and avoiding oversleeping may help normalize your sleep patterns and improve sleep quality over time

UNDERSTANDING NUTRIENT RATIOS

Keto macros are the most important aspect of the ketogenic diet. They include the three nutrients that your body needs in large amounts fat, protein, and carbs. Get them wrong and your chances of reaching ketosis are close to zero!

In this guide, we explain what macros are and how you can calculate your keto macros. We also offer practical bits of advice that can make meeting your keto macros a whole lot easier.

Calculating Keto Macros

The easiest way to calculate your keto macros is with a keto calculator. We've developed a precise keto calculator based on the standard ketogenic diet that will calculate you your keto macros in less than a minute. However, if you'd like to learn more about keto macros, including your daily allotment, keep reading.

What Are Macros?

Macros are nutrients that your body needs in large amounts in order to sustain wide range of metabolic processes. Medical and nutrition experts classify the following five nutrients as macros :

Carbohydrates

Proteins

Fats Fiber

Water

However, what most people refer to when talking about macros is carbohydrates, proteins, and fats. These three are also of great importance on a ketogenic diet. They are energy-providing nutrients whose total energy yield is defined in calories.

A balance in macros is also of huge importance for overall health. Studies show that eating too much or little of a single macro increases one's risk of obesity, heart disease, and diabetes. The worst offender of the three is carbs, but the one carrying the greatest stigma is fat (we'll talk more about that later).

Besides macronutrients, your body also needs micronutrients. Micronutrients are nutrients that you need to eat in smaller amounts, and they mostly include vitamins and minerals. It's easy to get adequate amounts of both micro and macronutrients from a well-planned ketogenic diet.

How to Calculate Macros For Keto

"Keto macros" is a term referring to the macronutrient ratio of a ketogenic diet. This ratio looks something like this:

60-75% of calories from fat

15-30% of calories from protein

5-10% of calories from carbs

This macronutrient ratio is different from what the medical community recommends and from what most people are used to. In fact, The Institute of Medicine recommends that active people get 45-65% of their energy from carbs, 10-35% from protein, and 20-35% from fat.

So, what's the deal here? Well, the goal of a keto diet is different from that of standard health diets. On a keto diet, your goal is to radically change the way your body uses nutrients for energy production by placing the body into a metabolic state called ketosis. The standard diet, on the other hand, is meant to optimize the way your body already makes and uses food for energy.

There are many reasons why you'd want to induce ketosis, but the most sought-after is to force your body to burn fat, instead of glucose, for fuel. When your body does this, you lose excess body fat, become more energized, and experience greater mental clarity.

Below is a breakdown of each macro so you can better understand their function on the keto diet:

Carbohydrates

Carbohydrates are your body's preferred fuel source. The reason for this is that they are easy to break down and turn into energy. However, unlike proteins and fat, carbs are still not an essential nutrient.

Carbs are simply a cheap and convenient sources of energy. In the absence of carbs, your body is perfectly adapted to surviving on protein and fats. Not only that, but your body may just benefit from occasional carb restriction.

The biggest problem with carbs is that they're easy to overconsume. The typical Western diet is laden with all of the wrong carbs, and this is believed to be behind the global rise in metabolic diseases and obesity.

Another problem with carbs is that some can cause low-grade inflammation, a condition linked to things like cancer and cardiovascular diseases.

The keto diet minimizes carb intake to a level that will help your body burn fat and also maintain good health.

Protein

Protein is an essential macronutrient that the body needs to build and repair tissue. Proteins are large molecules consisting of amino acids. There are around 20 amino acids in nature, 9 of which are essential for human health. You can get essential amino acids from both plant and animal foods.

On a keto diet, you have to adjust your protein intake in accordance with your activity levels: the more active you are, the more protein you'll need. However, going overboard on protein can, and will, kick you out of ketosis because your body is able to turn a portion of the protein you eat into glucose.

On a positive note, one great thing about protein is that it keeps you feeling full for a long time because it takes longer to digest. Protein also boosts weight loss because your body actually burns calories to digest it. Finally, protein builds muscle tissue, which further increases your energy expenditure.

Fats

Fat is a central keto macro but also the reason behind much of today's nutrition controversy. Medical experts have been warning the public about the dangers of high-fat diets for decades. The fact of the matter is that fat is an essential nutrient that your body cannot do without. Eliminating it from your diet does more harm than good, and researchers have been saying this for at least two decades now after reevaluating the role of fat in health and disease.

What we now know about fat is that it:

Provides energy

Helps your body use fat-soluble vitamins (A, D, E, and K)

Maintains body temperature

Maintains healthy skin and hair Promotes

cell health

Accumulates toxins to protect internal organs

Supports hormone production

Fat is central to the ketogenic diet, helping the body make ketones to fuel your body and brain by replacing glucose. If you lower your calorie intake, your body will also start to use stored fat for energy.

Types of Fat

There are many different types of fat, some good and some bad.

Bad fats are trans fats found in excess in highly processed and fried food. Some margarines are also high in trans fats. Good fats are the monounsaturated and polyunsaturated fats found in plant oils. Saturated fats are also good, but some may not agree with this. Keto experts vouch for it as do many researchers and medical experts today.

Fats also contain essential and non-essential fatty acids. Essential fatty acids are alpha-linolenic acid (omega-3 fatty acids) and linoleic acid (omega-6 fatty acids). Your body can make other fatty acids from omega fats, but it cannot make omega fats on its own so you need to get them from food.

You can get essential fatty acids from a wide range of food sources. The best sources by far are fish, other seafood, nuts, plant oils, and seeds. Eating a variety of these foods is a foolproof way to meet your daily needs for omega fatty acids.

How to Calculate Macros for Keto

Keto macros are roughly the same for your most people. However, for maximum efficiency, you want keto macros to match your physique, needs, and goals. The easiest way to do that is by using a keto calculator.

However, there are other ways to calculate and keep track of your keto macros:

1. Start with net carbs

Net carbs are total carbs minus fiber. Calculating them is important on a keto diet because your body makes glucose only from net carbs. Fiber has no effect on your blood glucose levels whatsoever, so feel free to load up on it.

Take a look at nutrition labels on food packaging or online for fresh produce.

Your daily intake of net carbs should not exceed 30 grams. This is the upper limit you can reach before being kicked out of ketosis. However, eating around 20 grams a day is optimal for most people. Athletes may need to eat more to have enough energy during workouts.

2. Move on to proteins

Your protein allowance on a keto diet will depend on whether you want to build muscle, lose weight, and your body fat percentage*. As a rule of thumb, you need around 1.5 to 2.5 grams of protein per kilogram of muscle mass to maintain or gain muscle**. That's 0.7 to 1 grams of protein per pound of muscle mass. You will need less if you are not trying to gain muscle. Below is a formula to help you determine your daily protein allowance.

a) Start by calculating your body fat by using the following formula (the example provided is for someone weighing 160 pounds with a 20 % body fat percentage):

160 pounds x 0.20 (20 %) = 32 pounds of body fat

b) Subtract your body fat percentage from 100 to get your lean muscle mass percentage: 100 - 20 percent (of body fat) = 80% of muscle mass

c) Then divide this by 100 to get the decimal for your muscle weight: 80 / 100 = 0.80

d) Finally, multiply this decimal by total weight to calculate your total lean mass weight: 160 (pounds) x 0.80 = 128 of lean mass

e) To calculate your daily protein allowance, simply multiply your muscle mass by gram of protein. The formula goes like this:

128 pounds (of muscle mass) x 0.7-1 grams (protein per pound of muscle mass) = 89- 128 grams of protein

3. Finish with fats

After you've determined your daily carb and protein allowance, you'll have to calculate how much fat you should eat. This will depend on whether you want to lose or maintain weight. To maintain weight, you need to eat more fat than to lose weight.

The easiest way to calculate your daily fat allowance is, of course, by using a keto calculator. The calculator will provide you with your daily allowance of fat in grams. If you want to know how many calories you are taking in, consider the following facts:

Protein and carbohydrates contain 4 calories per gram Fat

contains 9 calories per gram.

This means that if, say, a keto (macros) calculator shows you need to eat 200 grams of fat that 1,800 of your daily calories should come from fat:

200 grams (of fat) x 9 calories (per gram) = 1,800 calories from fat

On average, women need to eat around 2,000 and men around 2,500 calories per day. But these numbers vary greatly depending on your age, weight, and physical activity levels along with your goals (if you're trying to lose weight or gain muscle mass).

A surplus of 500 calories will either help you maintain muscle mass or total weight, while a deficiency will help you lose body fat. However, we need to mention that many keto experts doubt the necessity of counting calories on a keto diet. The reason being that fat is highly satiating, so going overboard is difficult. Another reason is that the ketogenic diet in itself suppresses appetite [8] but also has a strong thermic effect.

How to Calculate Food Macros

You know that some foods are high in fat and low in carbs, while others are the exact opposite (think avocado vs. white rice). But that doesn't really help you on a practical level. You want to know how many keto macros you're taking in with your meals.

Calculating keto macros in food items as well as whole meals is pretty easy. However, we need to warn you that it can be time-consuming when you first start doing this. Nevertheless, calculating macros is an important step in getting your ratio just right. You can do this by using nutrition facts from reliable websites.

Take for example Myfitnesspal.com. The website offers nutrition facts for a wide range of food items. Simply enter a food item in the search bar and the website will give you precise nutrition facts per serving, including total fat, total carbs, dietary fiber, protein, and calories.

Besides Myfitnesspal.com, you can use our food list of keto-approved foods and visit our Foods & Nutrition Blogs to learn more about keto foods. Once you have a list of keto foods ready, use nutrition facts websites to calculate your keto macros.

Example:

1 medium avocado (250 calories)

Fat: 23 grams

Net carbs: 5 grams (15 grams total carbs - 10 grams fiber),

Protein: 0 grams

Served with one poached egg (74 calories)

Fat: 5 grams

Net carbs: 0 grams

Protein: 6 grams

Topped with a teaspoon of olive oil (40 calories)

Fat: 5 grams

Net carbs: 0 grams

Protein: 0 grams

From this 364-calorie meal, you get a total of 33 grams of fat, 5 grams of net carbs, and 6 grams of protein. Make similar lists for all your meals and keep them close when you plan your meals.

Tips & Tricks for Meeting Macros

Stick to whole foods

Highly processed foods contain hidden ingredients that can sabotage your dieting efforts. In other words, you never know what you are taking in when munching on packaged foods labeled "low-carb" or "keto". The keto diet is all about clean eating as this supports good health, and most importantly – helps you stay within your keto macros.

Plan your meals

Planning meals is non-negotiable on a keto diet. You simply can't make food choices on spur of the moment because then you won't be able to track your keto macros. Planning meals is time-consuming at first. But once you have your list ready, most of your planning is already done.

Find a ready-made meal plan

An even easier way to meet your keto macros is to use existing meal plans. Many keto websites offer weekly, monthly, and even half-year meal plans. This takes away much of the hassle that you initial go through when trying to plan meals and meet keto macros. Make sure you only use meal plans from reputable sources with good ratings.

Take-Home Message

Keto macros are the essence of a ketogenic diet. You want to balance them out perfectly to reach your goals and feel good along the way. This can be a bit tricky as it involves plenty of planning and mathematics.

But once you have your macros set and your meal plan in place, keto dieting will become your second nature. Use our keto calculator, read our informative blog posts, and consider our guidance and tips given here when trying to meet your macros.

DANGERS OF EATING KETO

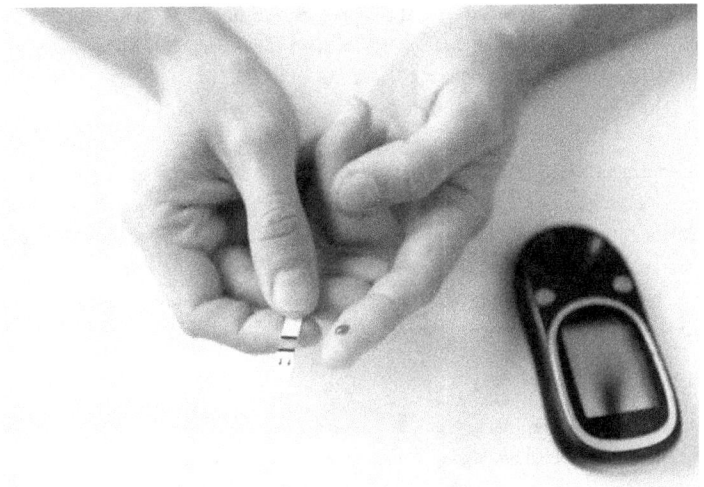

Here are some potential challenges and dangers of eating keto.

1.   Athletic Performance Impediments: For those people who train heavy and hard, going keto might cramp your style. As important as protein is for muscle growth, carbs also play an equally critical role by releasing insulin to drive that protein into muscles faster. It also helps us build up glycogen stores for longer training sessions, runs or hikes. One comprehensive review of the literature in sports nutrition found that while research is lacking on the long-term impacts of the keto diet, in the short term, the keto diet is inferior to other diet protocols on anaerobic, aerobic and in some cases even strength performance measures.

2. Keto "Flu": Your body isn't accustomed to using ketones on the regular, so when you make the switch, you tend to feel unwell. The keto diet also influences electrolyte balance, resulting in brain fog, headaches, nausea and fatigue. Keto dieters also consistently complain about getting bad-smelling breath, sweat and pee as a result of the by-product of fat metabolism (acetone) seeping out. Thankfully, this effect is just temporary, so just know you won't have to spend your life smelling rank.

3. Constipation: No one likes to feel backed up, and sadly if you're not careful about your diet choices when going keto, it could become a regular concern. One 10-year (albeit small) study looking at the effects of a keto diet on young children found that 65 percent experienced digestive woes. Thankfully, going keto is not a life sentence for problem bowels. Since you're cutting out whole grains and fruit (two of the most common sources of fiber), aim to up your fiber-rich veggies, and consider a supplement.

4. Nutrition Deficiencies: As with any super-restrictive regimen, when you cut food out, there's a good chance you'll be missing something big. Here's what you need to keep an eye open for.

5. Sodium: Believe it or not, depending on your diet, you may be low on salt. When carb intake is low and insulin isn't being excreted, the kidneys absorb less sodium and potassium and excrete more as waste, leaving you feeling dizzy, fatigued and grumpy. Rather than reaching for more processed food, try seasoning your food a little more liberally with sea salt.

6. Potassium: With the approved list of foods being so brief, you might not be getting in enough fruits and veggies on keto. One of the biggest impacts? A potassium deficiency— and all of the lovely constipation and muscle cramps that accompanies it. Aim to up

your intake of foods like spinach, avocado, tomatoes, kale and mushrooms to get your potassium fix.

7.   Vitamin C: Most of our vitamin C intake comes from a nice array of fruits, so if you're cutting all of that out, you'll have to make sure you're keeping your veggies up to compensate. Reach for more broccoli, Brussels sprouts, cauliflower and cabbage to ensure you get your fill.

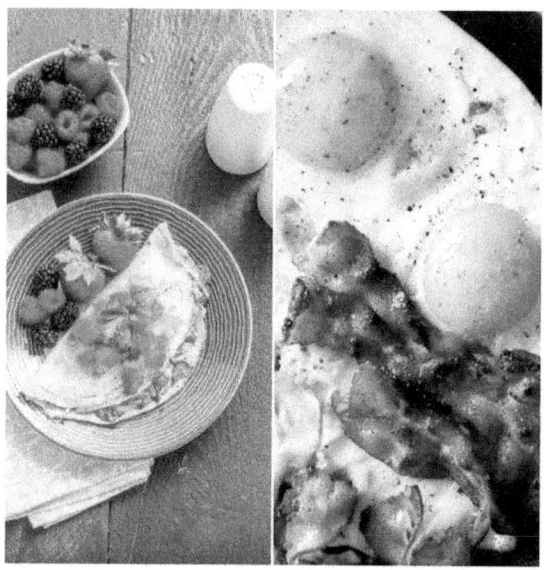

Obesity rivals smoking as the number one cause of preventable death. One reason is the dramatic rise in the diabetes risk often accompanying weight gain. So, are you interested in starting up a new diet plan, one aimed to not only help you lose weight but to control your blood sugar better? Chances are you are searching for the best options available. Two you may come across as they are trendy in today's times are the ketogenic diet and the paleo diet. Many people actually get confused between these as they do tend to be similar so it can be hard to differentiate between them.

Let us compare so you can see which one is right for you...

Carb Sources. First, let's talk carb sources as this is where the two diets vastly differ...

with the paleo diet plan, your carb sources are going to be any fresh fruit, along with sweet potatoes. Together, you can quickly achieve 100 grams or more of carbohydrates between these two foods.

the keto diet, on the other hand, your only carb source is leafy greens, and even those are restricted.

So one of the most significant differences between the ketogenic diet and the paleo diet plan is the ketogenic diet is deficient in carbohydrates while the paleo is not. You can make the paleo diet very low carb if you want, but it is not by default. There is more flexibility in food choices.

Calorie Counting. Next, we come to calorie counting. This is also a place where the two diets differ considerably.

With the keto diet, you will be calorie and macro counting quite heavily. You need to hit specific targets...

30% total protein intake, 5%

carbohydrate intake and 65%

dietary fat intake.

If you do not reach these targets, you are not going to move into the "state of ketosis," which is the entire point of this diet plan.

With the paleo diet, there are no strict rules around this. While you can count calories if you want, you do not have to. Obviously, your fat loss results will likely be better if you do monitor calories to some degree since calories do dictate whether you gain or lose body fat, but it is not essential.

Exercise Fuel Availability. Which brings us to our next point - exercise fuel availability. To be able to exercise with intensity, you need carbohydrates in your diet plan. You cannot get fuel availability if you are not eating carbohydrate-rich foods - that means the keto diet is not going to support intense exercise sessions. For this reason, the keto diet will not be optimal for most people. Exercise is an integral part of staying healthy, so it is strongly recommended you exercise and do not follow a diet that limits exercise.

Of course, you can do the targeted ketogenic diet or the cyclic ketogenic diet, both of which have you including carbohydrates in the diet at some point...

the targeted ketogenic diet has you eating carbohydrates just before starting your workout session while

the cyclic ketogenic diet calls for you to eat a larger dose of carbs over the weekend, which are designed to sustain you through the rest of the week.

If you follow either of these, you can choose any carbohydrates you wish; it does not necessarily have to be just sweet potatoes or fruit.

There you have some critical differences between this two approaches...

the ketogenic diet is one focusing more on tracking macros and is intended to assist with fat loss while

the paleo diet focuses more on good food choices and health and hopes weight loss comes as a result.

Although managing Type 2 diabetes can be very challenging, it is not a condition you must just live with. Make simple changes to your daily routine - include exercise to help lower both your blood sugar levels and your weight.

Does A Keto Diet Help Lower Blood Sugar Levels

Is a ketogenic diet safe for people who have received a diagnosis of Type 2 diabetes? The food recommended for people with high blood sugar encourages weight loss: a ketogenic diet has high amounts of fat and is low in carbs, so it is mystifying how such a high-fat diet is an option for alleviating high blood sugar.

The ketogenic diet underlines a low intake of carbohydrates and increased consumption of fat and protein. The body then breaks down fat by a process called "ketosis," and produces a source of fuel called ketones. Usually, the diet improves blood sugar levels while decreasing the body's need for insulin. The diet initially was developed for epilepsy treatment, but the kinds of food and the eating pattern it highlights, are being studied for the benefit of those with Type 2 diabetes.

The ketogenic diet contains foods such as... pasta,

fruits, and bread

as a source of body energy. People with Type 2 diabetes suffer from high and unstable blood sugar levels, and the keto diet helps them by allowing the body to preserve their blood sugar at a low healthy level.

How does a keto diet help many with Type 2 diabetes? In 2016, the Journal of Obesity and Eating Disorders published a review suggesting a keto diet may help people with diabetes by improving their A1c test results, more than a calorie diet.

The ketogenic diet places emphasis on the consumption of more protein and fat, making you feel less hungry and therefore leading to weight loss. Protein and fat take longer to digest than carbohydrates and helps to keep energy levels up.

In a nutshell, the ketogenic diet... lowers

blood sugar,

enhances insulin sensitivity and

promotes less dependency on medications.

The Keto Diet Plan. Ketogenic diets are stringent, but if adhered to correctly they can provide a nourishing and healthful nutrition routine. It is about staying away from carbohydrate foods likely to spike blood sugar levels.

People with Type 2 diabetes are often advised to focus on this diet plan as it consists of a mix of low carbohydrate foods, high-fat content, and moderate protein. It is also important because it avoids high-processed foods and indulges in lightly processed and healthy foods.

A ketogenic diet should consist of these types of food...

low-carb vegetables: eat vegetables with every meal. Avoid starchy vegetables like corn and potatoes.

eggs: they contain a low amount of carbohydrates and are a high source of protein.

meats: eat fatty meats but avoid excessive amounts. High amounts of protein plus low carbohydrates can lead to the liver converting protein into glucose, thus causing the person to come out of ketosis.

fish: an excellent source of protein.

Eat from healthy sources of fat like avocados, seeds, nuts, and olive oil.

Although managing your disease can be very challenging, Type 2 diabetes is not a condition you must just live with. You can make simple changes to your daily routine and lower both your weight and your blood sugar levels. Hang in there, the longer you do it, the easier it gets.

Should You Use A Ketogenic Diet Plan

As someone who is working hard to control or prevent Type 2 diabetes, one diet you may have heard about is the ketogenic or keto diet plan. This diet is a very low carbohydrate diet plan consisting of around...

5% total carbohydrates, 30%

protein, and a whopping 65%

dietary fat.

If there is one thing this diet will do, its help to control your blood sugar levels. This said, there is more to eating well than just controlling your blood sugar.

Let's go over some of the main reasons why this diet doesn't always stack up to be as great as it sounds...

1. You'll Be Lacking Dietary Fiber. The first big problem with the ketogenic diet is you'll be seriously lacking in dietary fiber. Almost all vegetables are cut from this plan (apart from the very low-carb varieties), and fruits are definitely not permitted. High fiber grains are also out of the equation, so this leaves you with primarily protein and fats - two foods containing no fiber at all.

2. You'll Be Low In Energy. Another big issue with the ketogenic diet is you'll be low in energy to carry out your exercise program. Your body can only utilize glucose as a fuel source for very intense exercise and if you aren't taking in carbohydrates, you'll have no glucose available.

3. You May Suffer Brain Fog. Those who are using the ketogenic diet may also find they suffer from brain fog. Again, this is thanks to the fact your brain primarily runs off glucose.

4. Your Antioxidant Status Will Decline. Finally, the last issue with the ketogenic diet is due to the lack of fruit and vegetable content - your antioxidant status is going to sharply decline.

So keep these points in mind as the diet comes with some risks. The ketogenic diet converts fat instead of sugar into energy. It was first created as a treatment for epilepsy but now the effects of the diet are being looked at to help Type 2 diabetics lower their blood sugar. Make sure you discuss the diet with your doctor before making any dietary chan

RELATIONSHIP BETWEEN DIABETES AND KETOACIDOSIS

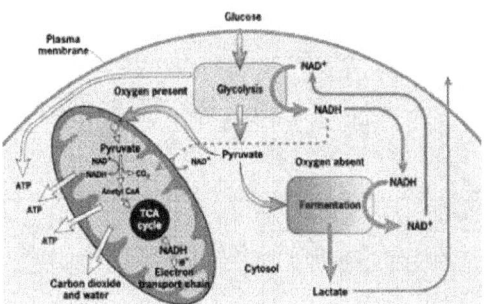

For those with type 1 diabetes, ketoacidosis is a common, severe complication. Diabetic ketoacidosis occurs when the blood is very acidic and the blood glucose levels are very high.

The prefix "keto" refers to the substance known in the body as "ketones." Ketones are created by your body during the process of breaking down of fat. When the levels of ketones in the blood stream get really high the blood becomes very acidic.

In many cases, it is the acid blood that first indicates to doctors that a patient may have type 1 diabetes. If the doctors already know you have type 1 diabetes, they are not so surprised when you show symptoms of diabetic ketoacidosis in your tests. However, on average those with type 1 diabetes do not get diagnosed with ketoacidosis until they are at least 40 years old.

Ketoacidosis Is More Common in Type 1 Diabetics Than Type 2 Diabetics

People who have type 2 diabetes have reduced amounts of insulin production into their bloodstreams. People who have type 1 diabetes have dramatically reduced to know insulin production into their bloodstreams. This accounts for why those with type 1 diabetes are far more likely to develop ketoacidosis than those with type 2 diabetes.

Signs & Symptoms of Diabetic Ketoacidosis

1. Rapid Breathing

Your body may actually become acidic enough that it tries to use the lungs as a location to excrete acid. During this rapid breathing process, often referred to as "Kassmaul Breathing," your lungs are literally filled with acid from the bloodstream in a desperate attempt by your body to balance out the blood.

2. Nauseous Vomiting

As acids build up in your body it is very common to feel nauseous and to eventually begin vomiting. This may be another desperate attempt by your body to get rid of some acid. However, your bodily fluids may become very unbalanced, leading to further complications.

3. Chronic Drowsiness

The thick, acidic blood that gathers in the brain can cause you to become very drowsy and sluggish.

4. Weak Muscles

As ketoacidosis sets in your bloodstream will do an even worse job of distributing and using glucose where it is needed. As a result your muscles will not have the fuel they need to function the way they normally would. Every movement may seem like a chor

THE TRUTH ABOUT CARBS

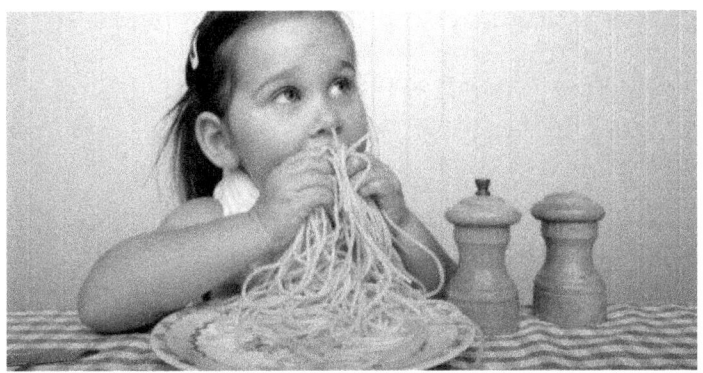

Carbohydrates are one of 3 macronutrients (nutrients that form a large part of our diet) found in food – the others being fat and protein.

Hardly any foods contain only 1 nutrient, and most are a combination of carbohydrates, fats and proteins in varying amounts.

There are 3 different types of carbohydrates found in food: sugar, starch and fibre.

Sugar

The type of sugars most adults and children in the UK eat too much of are called free sugars.

These are the sugars added to food or drinks, including sugars in biscuits, chocolate, flavoured yoghurts, breakfast cereals and fizzy drinks.

Sugars in honey, syrups (such as maple, agave and golden), nectars (such as blossom), and unsweetened fruit juices, vegetable juices and smoothies occur naturally, but still count as free sugars.

Sugar found naturally in milk, fruit and vegetables does not count.

Starch

Starch is found in foods that come from plants. Starchy foods, such as bread, rice, potatoes and pasta, provide a slow and steady release of energy throughout the day.

Fibre

Fibre is the name given to the diverse range of compounds found in the cell walls of foods that come from plants.

Good sources of fibre include vegetables with skins on, wholegrain bread, wholewheat pasta, and pulses (beans and lentils).

Why do we need carbs?

Carbohydrates are important to your health for a number of reasons.

Energy

Carbohydrates should be the body's main source of energy in a healthy, balanced diet, providing about 4kcal (17kJ) per gram.

They're broken down into glucose (sugar) before being absorbed into the bloodstream. From there, the glucose enters the body's cells with the help of insulin.

Glucose is used by your body for energy, fuelling all of your activities, whether going for a run or simply breathing.

Unused glucose can be converted to glycogen found in the liver and muscles.

If more glucose is consumed than can be stored as glycogen, it's converted to fat for long-term storage of energy.

Higher fibre starchy carbohydrates release sugar into the blood more slowly than sugary foods and drinks.

Disease risk

Fruit and vegetables, pulses, wholegrain and wholewheat varieties of starchy foods, and potatoes eaten with their skins on, are good sources of fibre.

Fibre is an important part of a healthy, balanced diet. It can promote good bowel health, reduce the risk of constipation, and some forms of fibre have been shown to reduce cholesterol levels.

Research shows diets high in fibre are associated with a lower risk of cardiovascular disease, type 2 diabetes and bowel cancer.

Many people don't get enough fibre. On average, most adults in the UK get about 19g of fibre a day. We're advised to eat an average of 30g a day.

Calorie intake

Carbohydrate contains fewer calories gram for gram than fat and starchy foods can be a good source of fibre, which means they can be a useful part of maintaining a healthy weight.

By replacing fatty, sugary foods and drinks with higher fibre starchy foods, it's more likely you'll reduce the number of calories in your diet.

Also, high-fibre foods add bulk to your meal, helping you feel full. "You still need to watch your portion sizes to avoid overeating," says Sian.

"Also watch the amount of fat you add when cooking and serving them: this increases the calorie content."

Should I cut out carbohydrates?

While we can most certainly survive without sugar, it would be quite difficult to eliminate carbohydrates entirely from your diet.

Carbohydrates are the body's main source of energy. In their absence, your body will use protein and fat for energy.

It may also be hard to get enough fibre, which is important for long-term health.

Healthy sources of carbohydrates, such as higher fibre starchy foods, vegetables, fruits and legumes, are also an important source of nutrients, such as calcium, iron and B vitamins.

Significantly reducing carbohydrates from your diet in the long term could put you at increased risk of insufficient intakes of certain nutrients, potentially leading to health problems.

Cutting out carbohydrates from your diet could put you at increased risk of a deficiency in certain nutrients, leading to health problems, unless you're able to make up for the nutritional shortfall with healthy substitutes.

Replacing carbohydrates with fats and higher fat sources of protein could increase your intake of saturated fat, which can raise the amount of cholesterol in your blood a risk factor for heart disease.

When you're low on glucose, the body breaks down stored fat to convert it into energy. This process causes a build-up of ketones in the blood, resulting in ketosis.

Ketosis as a result of a low-carbohydrate diet can be linked, at least in the short term, to headaches, weakness, nausea, dehydration, dizziness and irritability.

Try to limit the amount of sugary foods you eat and instead include healthier sources of carbohydrate in your diet, such as wholegrains, potatoes, vegetables, fruits, legumes and lower fat dairy products.

Don't protein and fat provide energy?

While carbohydrates, fat and protein are all sources of energy in the diet, the amount of energy each one provides varies:

carbohydrate provides: about 4kcal (17kJ) per gram protein

provides: 4kcal (17kJ) per gram

fat provides: 9kcal (37kJ) per gram

In the absence of carbohydrates in the diet, your body will convert protein (or other non-carbohydrate substances) into glucose, so it's not just carbohydrates that can raise your blood sugar and insulin levels.

If you consume more calories than you burn from whatever source, you'll gain weight.

So cutting out carbohydrates or fat doesn't necessarily mean cutting out calories if you're replacing them with other foods containing the same number of calories.

Are carbohydrates more filling than protein?

Carbohydrates and protein contain roughly the same number of calories per gram.

But other factors influence the sensation of feeling full, such as the type, variety and amount of food eaten, as well as eating behavior and environmental factors, like serving sizes and the availability of food choices.

The sensation of feeling full can also vary from person to person. Among other things, protein-rich foods can help you feel full, and we should have some beans, pulses, fish, eggs, meat and other protein foods as part of a healthy, balanced diet.

But we shouldn't eat too much of these foods. Remember that starchy foods should make up about a third of the food we eat and we all need to eat more fruit and vegetables.

How much carbohydrate should I eat?

The government's healthy eating advice, illustrated by the Eatwell Guide, recommends that just over a third of your diet should be made up of starchy foods, such as potatoes, bread, rice and pasta, and over another third should be fruit and vegetables.

This means that over half of your daily calorie intake should come from starchy foods, fruit and vegetables.

What carbohydrates should I be eating?

These are usually high in sugar and calories, which can increase the risk of tooth decay and contribute to weight gain if you eat them too often, while providing few other nutrients.

Fruit, vegetables, pulses and starchy foods (especially higher fibre varieties) provide a wider range of nutrients (such as vitamins and minerals), which are beneficial to health.

The fibre in these foods can help keep your bowels healthy and adds bulk to your meal, helping you feel full.

How can I increase my fibre intake?

To increase the amount of fibre in your diet, aim for at least 5 portions of a variety of fruit and veg a day.

Go for higher fibre varieties of starchy foods and eat potatoes with skins on. Try to aim for an average intake of 30g of fibre a day.

Here are some examples of the typical fibre content in some common foods: 2

breakfast wheat biscuits (approx. 37.5g) – 3.6g of fibre

1 slice of wholemeal bread – 2.5g (1 slice of white bread – 0.9g) 80g of

cooked wholewheat pasta – 4.2g

1 medium (180g) baked potato (with skin) – 4.7g

80g (4 heaped tablespoons) of cooked runner beans – 1.6g 80g

(3 heaped tablespoons) of cooked carrots – 2.2g

1 small cob (3 heaped tablespoons) of sweetcorn – 2.2g 200g

of baked beans – 9.8g

1 medium orange – 1.9g 1

medium banana – 1.4g

Can eating low glycaemic index (GI) foods help me lose weight?

The glycaemic index (GI) is a rating system for foods containing carbohydrates. It shows how quickly each food affects glucose (sugar) levels in your blood when that food is eaten on its own.

Some low-GI foods, such as wholegrain foods, fruit, vegetables, beans and lentils, are foods we should eat as part of a healthy, balanced diet.

But using GI to decide whether foods, or a combination of foods, are healthy or can help with weight reduction can be misleading.

Although low-GI foods cause blood sugar levels to rise and fall slowly, which may help you to feel fuller for longer, not all low-GI foods are healthy.

For example, watermelon and parsnips are high-GI foods, while chocolate cake has a lower GI value.

And the way a food is cooked and what you eat it with as part of a meal will change the GI rating.

This means GI alone isn't a reliable way of deciding whether foods, or combinations of foods, are healthy or will help you lose weight.

Do carbohydrates make you fat?

Any food can cause weight gain if you overeat. Whether your diet is high in fat or high in carbohydrates, if you frequently consume more energy than your body uses you're likely to put on weight.

In fact, gram for gram, carbohydrate contains fewer than half the calories of fat. Wholegrain varieties of starchy foods are good sources of fibre. Foods high in fibre add bulk to your meal and help you feel full.

But foods high in sugar are often high in calories, and eating these foods too often can contribute to you becoming overweight.

There's some evidence that diets high in sugar are associated with an increased energy content of the diet overall, which over time can lead to weight gain.

Can cutting out wheat help me lose weight?

Some people point to bread and other wheat-based foods as the main culprit for their weight gain.

Wheat is found in a wide range of foods, from bread, pasta and pizza to cereals and many other foods.

But there's not enough evidence that foods that contain wheat are any more likely to cause weight gain than any other food.

Unless you have a diagnosed health condition, such as wheat allergy, wheat sensitivity or coeliac disease, there's little evidence that cutting out wheat and other grains from your diet would benefit your health.

Grains, especially wholegrains, are an important part of a healthy, balanced diet.

Wholegrain, wholemeal and brown breads give us energy and contain B vitamins, vitamin E, fibre and a wide range of minerals.

White bread also contains a range of vitamins and minerals, but it has less fibre than wholegrain, wholemeal or brown breads.

If you prefer white bread, look for higher fibre options. Grains are also naturally low in fat.

Find out if cutting out bread could help ease bloating or other digestive symptoms

Should people with diabetes avoid carbs?

People with diabetes should try to eat a healthy, balanced diet, as shown in the Eatwell Guide.

They should also include higher fibre starchy foods at every meal. Steer clear of cutting out entire food groups.

It's recommended that everyone with diabetes sees a registered dietitian for specific advice on their food choices. Your GP can refer you to a registered dietitian.

There's some evidence that suggests low-carbohydrate diets can lead to weight loss and improvements in blood glucose control in people with type 2 diabetes in the short term.

But it's not clear whether the diet is a safe and effective way to manage type 2 diabetes in the long term.

Weight loss from a low-carbohydrate diet may be because of a reduced intake of calories overall and not specifically as a result of eating less carbohydrate.

There also isn't enough evidence to support the use of low-carbohydrate diets in people with type 1 diabetes.

What's the role of carbohydrates in exercise?

Carbohydrates, fat and protein all provide energy, but exercising muscles rely on carbohydrates as their main source of fuel.

But muscles have limited carbohydrate stores (glycogen) and need to be topped up regularly to keep your energy up.

A diet low in carbohydrates can lead to a lack of energy during exercise, early fatigue and delayed recovery.

When is the best time to eat carbohydrates?

There's little scientific evidence that one time is better than any other.

It's recommended that you base all your meals around starchy carbohydrate foods and you try to choose higher fibre wholegrain varieties when you can.

30 DAYS KETOGENIC DIET PLAN

WEEK1

In my eyes, simplicity is key for someone that is just starting out on a low carb diet. You don't want it to be a difficult transition (kitchen-wise), because it will be hard to just get rid of your cravings.

The first signs of ketosis are known as the "keto flu" where headaches, brain fogginess, fatigue, and the like can really rile your body up. Make sure that you're drinking plenty of waterand eating plenty of salt. The ketogenic diet is a natural diuretic and you'll be peeing more than normal. Take into account that you're peeing out electrolytes, and you can guess that you'll be having a thumping headache in no time. Keeping your salt intake and water intake high enough is very important, allowing your body to re-hydrate and re-supply your electrolytes. Doing this will help with the headaches, if not get rid of them completely.

If you need to, drink water with a sprinkling of salt in it. Just keep drinking water (I recommend 4 liters a day), and keep eating salt. It will help, trust me. If you're worried about high blood pressure and salt, don't be! Recent studies show that the sodium intake and blood pressure are not as correlated as we so once believed.

Breakfast.

For breakfast, you want to do something that's quick, easy, tasty, and of course – gives you leftovers. I suggest starting day 1 on a weekend. This way, you can make something that will last you for the entire week. The first week is all about simplicity. Nobody wants to be making breakfast before work, and we're not going to be doing that either!

Lunch.

We're also going to keep it simple here. Most of the time, it'll be salad and meat, slathered in high fat dressings and calling it a day. We don't want to get too rowdy here. You can use leftover meat from previous nights or use easy accessible canned chicken/fish. If you do use canned meats, try to read the labels and get the one that uses the least (or no) additives!

Dinner.

Dinner will be a combination of leafy greens (normally broccoli and spinach) with some meat. Again, we'll be going high on the fat and moderate on the protein.

P.S. No dessert for the first 2 weeks.

Week 2

Wow, week 1 is over. I hope you're still doing well on the diet and have found it pretty easy breezy to keep on track with everything!

This week we're going to be keeping it simple for breakfast again. We're going to introduce ketoproof coffee. It's a mixture of coconut oil, butter, and heavy cream in your coffee. If this repulses you – and I know some of you are saying "WHAT?" – just put some trust in me!

This concoction is not as strange as it sounds. Butter, after all, is made out of cream. So when you blend the oil, butter, and cream together it just adds a decadent richness to your coffee that I am quite sure you'll really like!

Breakfast.

For breakfast, we are going to change it up a bit. Here's where we introduce ketoproof coffee. Now, don't get me wrong – I know some of you won't like it. If you're not a fan of coffee, then try it with tea. If you're not a fan of the taste (which is very rare), then try making a mixture of the ingredients by themselves and eating it like that. So, why ketoproof coffee?

Fat Loss. Plain and simple, the consumption of medium-chain triglycerides (MCT) has been shown to lead to greater losses in adipose tissue (fat tissue), in both animals and humans.

Fats! Do I even need to explain this one? Eating fat has been shown to lead to greater amounts of energy, more efficient energy usage, and more effective weight loss. Not to mention, it's the main component of this diet.

More Energy. Studies have shown that the rapid rate of oxidation in MCFAs (Medium Chain Fatty Acids) leads to an increase in energy expenditure. Primarily, MCFAs are converted into ketones (our best friends), are absorbed differently in the body compared to regular oils, and give us more overall energy.

Feel free to add sweetener and spices to this if you're not the biggest fan of the taste. Cinnamon, stevia, vanilla extract. Whatever you'd like to make it great tasting. You can even switch up the taste each and every day so you don't get bored!

If this is your first time drinking ketoproof coffee, I suggest taking 1-2 hours or so to drink it down. Normally when people have a large exposure to coconut oil and they're not used to it, it can make them go to the bathroom quite often. Make sure you build a tolerance to coconut oil before drinking it within a 20 minute time frame.

Lunch.

We're still keeping simple here. We can incorporate more meat from the previous night of cooking into each lunch we do. Green vegetables and high fat dressings (or vinaigrettes) are key. Making sure to balance out the fats with the amounts of protein is very important.

Dinner.

Dinner, again, will be pretty simplistic. Meats, vegetables, high fat dressings are the center of our life. Maybe even a slathering of butter on our vegetables since we're getting friskier. Don't over think things in the first 2 weeks; simple is success.

P.S. No dessert for this week either, but we'll be delving into that next week!

Week 3

This week we're introducing a slight fast. We're going to get full on fats in the morning and fast all the way until dinner time. Not only are there a myriad of health benefits to this, it's also easier on our eating schedule (and cooking schedule). I suggest eating (rather, drinking) your breakfast at 7am and then eating dinner at 7pm. Keeping 12 hours between your 2 meals. This will help put your body into a fasted state.

In a fasting state, our bodies can break down extra fat that's stored for the energy it needs. When we're in ketosis, our body already mimics a fasting state, being that we have little to no glucose in our bloodstream, so we use the fats in our bodies as energy.

Intermittent fasting is using the same reasoning – instead of using the fats we are eating to gain energy, we are using our stored fat. That being said, you might think it's great – you can just fast and lose more weight. You have to take into account that later on, you will need to eat extra fat in order to keep out of a starvation mode state.

There are a number of benefits shown that come from intermittent fasting. Some of these include blood lipid levels, longevity, and the much needed mental clarity.

If you find that you can't do a fast, then no big deal. Go back to week 1 and experiment as you see fit. You can eat what you want as long as it fits into your macros.

This is where things start to get more fun – less to worry about, more deliciousness to cook!

Breakfast.

We're going full on fats with breakfast, just like we did last week. This time we'll double the amount of ketoproof coffee (or tea) we drink, meaning we double the amount of coconut oil, butter, and heavy cream. It should come to quite a lot of calories, and should definitely keep us full all the way to dinner. Remember to continue drinking water like a fiend to make sure you're staying hydrated.

Lunch.

No lunch, oh no! Don't worry – the fats from the morning should keep you feeling energized and full all the way through lunch. Normally people start hitting a wall at first at around 2pm, so make sure you have plenty of water to drink, drink, and drink.

Dinner.

Well, dinner is staying the same. Meats, vegetables, and fats are almost always going to be the dinnertime norm. But don't worry – we'll mix in some bread-y type things!

And guess what, we get to eat dessert this week! Woo! We'll be creating some low carb and great tasting treats that will reward you ever so much for doing the fasting. Sweets, treats, and losing weight lucky us, right?

Week 4

This week we're getting stricter with our fasting. We had a full week of intermittent fasting and now we're going to skip breakfast and lunch. Water is our BEST friend here! Don't forget that you can drink coffee, tea, flavored water, and the like to get your liquids in. Keep drinking to make sure you're not thinking about your stomach. It MIGHT start growling, just ignore it – your body will adjust with time.

Now, if you're the kind of person that can't fast then you can go back and follow week 2 again. That's no big deal. Though fasting does take some time for the body to get used to, so I suggest putting your best efforts into it. Not only are the health benefits fantastic, the self-control that you gain from doing so is really a great thing.

This is by far my favorite week because it most closely resembles how I eat on a daily basis. I normally set a window of 6 hours for myself to eat in. From waking up until 5pm, I fast. After that, I am open to eating until 11pm. This is where the real fun begins. Eating copious amounts of food and being full all the way through the next day.

You get to start experimenting more with dessert and dinner. You get to snack as you please inside your window and best of all – you get to eat that protein laden chicken that you've been missing so much of!

Breakfast.

We're fasting! Black coffee if you're a caffeine addict like me. Tea, if you are not into the coffee so much. Tea can add great health benefits like coffee also. Some of the great benefits of green tea are:

Polyphenols – These function as antioxidants in your body. The most powerful antioxidant in green tea is Epigallocatechin gallate (EGCG), which has shown to be effective against fatigue.

Improved Brain Function – Not only does green tea contain caffeine, it also contains L-theanine, which is an amino acid. L-theanine increases your GABA activity, which improves anxiety, dopamine, and alpha waves.

Increased Metabolic Rate – Green tea has been shown to improve your metabolic rate. In combination with the caffeine, this can lead up to 15% increased fat oxidization.

Lunch.

Water, water, and then some more water. You don't get to eat lunch and you don't get to eat breakfast. So make sure you keep yourself VERY hydrated. It's imperative here that you do a good job with your hydration. Remember – I recommend 4 liters a day.

Dinner.

Lots and lots of food with dessert to cover the bases! Dinner is a fantastic time for me. I suggest breaking your fast with a small snack, then after 30-45 minutes eat to your hearts content. Normally I need 2 meals to get to my macros, and I think you'll need to do the same.

Week 5

This is where we have to depart! Sorry to say but you're on your own. You should have plenty of leftovers that are frozen, ready, and waiting! I know a lot of you out there have trouble with timing and are busy people so making sure that some nights you make extras to freeze is important. All those leftovers you have in the freezer? Use them up. Create your own meal plan, at first using this as a guide, and then completely doing it yourself. Once you get the hang of it, it'll be a sinch – I promise you!!

IN CONCLUSION

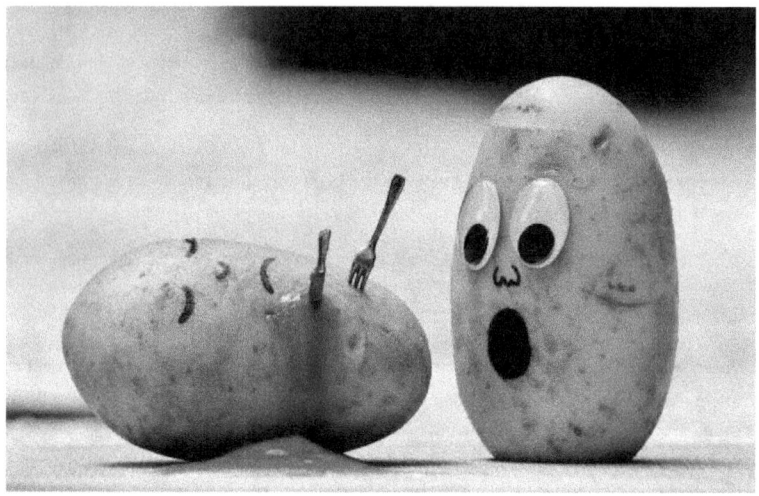

Eating a high amount of fat, moderate protein, and low amount of carbs can have a massive impact on your health lowering your cholesterol, body weight, blood sugar, and raising your energy and mood levels.

A ketogenic diet can be hard to fathom in the beginning but isn't as hard as it's made out to be. The transition can be a little bit tough, but the growing popularity of the clean eating movement makes it easier and easier to find available low-carb foods.

Keep it straightforward and strict. You usually see better results in people who restrict their carb intake further. Try to keep your carbs as low as possible for the first month of keto. Keep it strict by cutting out excess sweets and artificial sweeteners altogether (like diet soda). Cutting these out dramatically decreases sugar cravings.

Drink water and supplement electrolytes. Most common problems come from dehydration or lack of electrolytes. When you start keto (and even in the long run), make sure that you drink plenty of water, salt your foods, and take a multivitamin. If you're still experiencing issues, you can order electrolyte supplements individually.

Track what you eat. It's so easy to over-consume on carbs when they're hidden in just about everything you pick up. Keeping track of what you eat helps control your carb intake and keep yourself accountable.

Anti-Inflammatory Diet For Beginners

Table of Contents

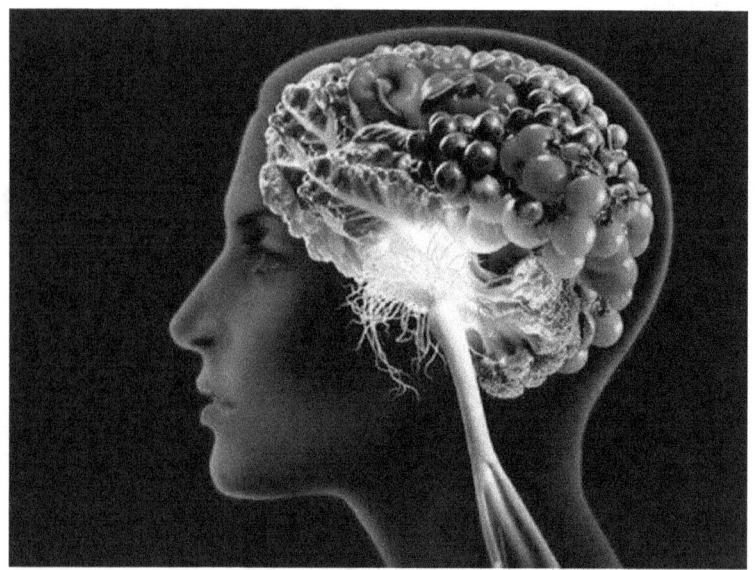

One of the most incredible and complex parts of the human body is the immune system. The immune system is able to recognize foreign substances like viruses and bacteria that might do our body harm.

It's important to know that there are two main parts of the immune system. The first is innate immunity and you are born with it totally intact; its job is to protect you against outside threats through its protective barriers like mucus and stomach acid. Fevers and the cough reflex are some other example of antigens that the innate immunity handles.

The second type of immunity makes up the adaptive immune system and it's constantly developing as you develop in life. Each time you are exposed to a germ or illness, your adaptive immune system keeps a record of it and helps your body build up a pre-programmed defense. And then, ideally, it won't make you sick the next time you come into contact with it. This adaptive immune process involves a complex system of chemicals, cells, and biological pathways that make up one of the great wonders of the human body.

The immune system and inflammation go hand in hand, and causing an inflammatory response is one major way the immune system responds to a threat and starts to fight off bacteria or tissue damage.

WHAT IS INFLAMMATION

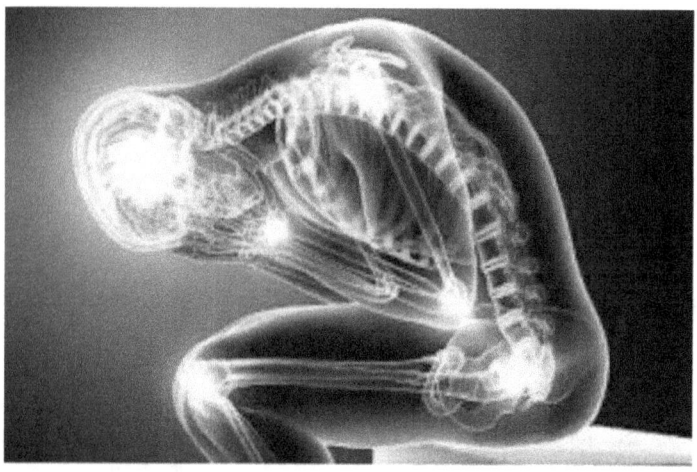

Inflammation is a natural process with the biological purpose to initiate healing by increasing circulation. It is a complex process involving both the immune system and vascular system and the interplay of various chemical mediators. Increased circulation brings white blood cells and nourishment to the site of injury or infection so that invading pathogens are killed and damage may be repaired. Characteristic signs of inflammation include pain (dolor), heat (calor), swelling (tumor) and redness (rubor).

When Inflammation Goes Awry:

While some inflammation is beneficial and appropriate for healing, chronic or excessive inflammation, serving no purpose produces damage. Chronic inflammation has a bad reputation because it is implicated in various disease processes including (but not limited to)...

- autoimmune diseases

- arthritis

- diabetes

- Alzheimer's disease

- atherosclerosis (hardening of arteries that leads to heart attack and stroke)

- ADD and ADHD

- allergies & asthma

- cancers

- inflammatory bowel disease

Soft tissue swelling and chemical mediators involved in inflammation can also irritate nerve endings, contributing to pain.

What is the Anti-Inflammatory Diet?

It is a well-known fact that different foods are metabolized differently, some promoting inflammation and others reducing it. The purpose of the anti-inflammatory diet is to promote optimal health and healing by choosing foods that reduce inflammation. If one can successfully control excessive inflammation through natural means (like through diet), it reduces one's dependence on anti-inflammatory medications that have unwanted and unhealthy side effects and don't solve the underlying problem. While anti-inflammatory medications (such as NSAIDs) is a quick fix to ease symptoms, they ultimately weaken the immune system by damaging the gastrointestinal tract which plays an important role in immune system function.

Anti-inflammatory Diet Basics:

In general, eat an abundance of fresh vegetables and fruits, whole grains, anti-inflammatory fats and nuts while limiting processed foods, meat protein, milk products, refined sugars, artificial colors/flavors/sweeteners and food sensitivities.

Vegetables:

Enjoy an abundance of fresh vegetables and fruits in a variety of colors (preferably organic). Fruits and vegetables are full of vitamins, minerals, antioxidants and fiber which give the body the essential building blocks for health. Examples include beans, squash, lintels, sweet potatoes, cruciferous vegetables, avocados, dark leafy greens... There are so many choices! As for fruits, pineapple and papaya are particularly good because they are high in bromelain, a powerful natural anti-inflammatory. Fruits and vegetables also make great, healthy snacks.

Avoid / Limit:

Avoid produce that is not grown organically. Toxic chemical residues from herbicides and pesticides can remain and when ingested are foreign irritants to the system. Many crops in North America are also genetically engineered and are put on the market without rigorous scientific study to determine safety for human consumption. Independent research is finally being done to show toxic effects of consuming genetically modified organisms. Foreign DNA is randomly inserted into the genome of a crop. Examples include herbicide resistant corn and soy which are resistant to the herbicide Roundup, made by Monsanto. Roughly 90% of all corn and soy sold in North America is genetically modified. Also be aware of derivatives of genetically modified ingredients (such as corn starch and corn syrup etc.). It has also been suggested that consuming GMOs is a contributing factor to the rise in allergies as our bodies are recognizing these food substances as foreign. By choosing items with the "certified organic" label, you avoid both GMOs and toxic herbicides/pesticides.

For some people, vegetables in the nightshade family may pose a concern. Examples of nightshade vegetables include tomatoes, peppers, potatoes and eggplant. Nightshades contain alkaloids which are thought to exacerbate inflammation and joint damage in certain susceptible individuals with arthritis (though research is conflicting). Thus, for some individuals, limiting or avoiding nightshade vegetables may be beneficial.

Fats:

Enjoy healthy, anti-inflammatory fats including olive oil, coconut oil, avocados, nuts, salmon and sardines. In humans, there are two essential fatty acids, alpha-linolenic acid (an omega-3) and linoleic acid (an omega-6). These are "essential" because they are required for good health but the body does not synthesize them. Omega-3 fats are anti-inflammatory. Omega-6 fats can be pro-inflammatory or anti-inflammatory (as it can be metabolized by two different pathways). Researchers suggest that keeping the ratio of omega-6 to omega-3 between 2:1 and 4:1 is best for health. The modern diet tends to be high in omega-6 as it is abundantly available in cooking oils. Thus, including rich sources of omega-3 is important (such as fish, flax and walnuts especially).

Avoid / Limit:

Fats to limit or avoid include margarine, butter, shortening, hydrogenated oils, trans fats, saturated fats, and milk fat. Omega-6 fats are very high in corn oil, safflower oil and sunflower oil. Trans fats are linked with inflammatory diseases.

Meat:

In general, limit animal proteins because they tend to acidify the body and also promote inflammation. When selecting animal protein, enjoy fish, poultry (especially free-range and organically raised), lamb and omega-3 eggs.

Avoid / Limit:

Limit beef, pork, shellfish and factory farmed eggs. In general, grass-fed is superior to grain-fed. Avoid charred foods, smoked foods and cold cuts. Cold cuts contain nitrates and nitrites which promote cancer. Barbequed foods contain polycyclic aromatic hydrocarbons (PAHs) and heterocyclic amines (HCAs) which also promote cancer.

Dairy:

Enjoy dairy substitutes in moderation (such as almond milk).

Avoid / Limit:

Avoid or limit dairy products in general. This includes milk, yogurt, cheese and ice cream. As we age, we lose the enzyme that digests dairy, resulting in lactose intolerance and inflammation. The milk protein, casein, is also acidifying which (despite what many people are brought up thinking) robs the bones of calcium.

Grains:

Enjoy whole grains as opposed to refined grains. Refined grains are grains in which the germ and bran have been removed. This means there is loss of fiber, minerals and vitamins. In other words, the good stuff is removed in exchange for a longer shelf life. Some good examples of healthy grains include (organic) whole wheat/oats/bulgar/coucous, quinoa and whole oats (like steel-cut oats).

Whole grains are also a rich source of complex carbohydrates. Complex carbohydrates (as opposed to simple sugars) will prevent spikes in your blood sugar level. Sugar promotes inflammation.

Avoid / Limit:

Avoid or limit refined carbohydrates such as white bread, pastries, sweet things and pastas.

Nuts:

Enjoy nuts and nut butters such as almonds, walnuts, sesame seeds, pumpkin seeds and flax.

Avoid / Limit:

Avoid any specific nut allergies.

Beverages:

Enjoy plenty of pure, filtered water (avoiding chlorine, fluoride and other contaminants which are irritants that promote inflammation). Other great choices are lemon water and herbal teas.

Avoid / Limit:

Avoid sugary sodas, fruit juice (with sugar added) and milk.

Spices:

Many spices reduce inflammation. Some great examples are turmeric, oregano, rosemary, ginger, garlic and cinnamon. Bioflavenoids and polyphenols reduce inflammation and fight free radicals. Cayenne pepper is also anti-inflammatory, as it contains capsicum. Capsicum is often used in pain-relief creams.

Sweeteners:

Enjoy stevia, molasses, maple syrup or honey as better alternatives for refined sugar.

Avoid / Limit:

Avoid refined sugar, fructose and especially high fructose corn syrup which promote inflammation. Avoid artificial sweeteners.

Other:

Enjoy fermented foods such as kimchi, miso soup and sauerkraut. Fermented foods are probiotic and help to rebuild the immune system by supporting healthy microflora in the gut and to reduce inflammation. Fermented foods also tend to be easy to digest and are also factories for B vitamins.

Avoid / Limit:

In general, eliminate processed foods, artificial colors, artificial flavors and preservatives. Also avoid foods that you have a known sensitivity or allergy to as this promotes inflammation. Low grade sensitivities are easy to miss, so if you're unsure, have a food allergy test. Some of the most common problem foods include wheat (gluten), corn, soy, milk and nuts.

Everything we need for health, can be found in nature. We just need to choose well. If you need help and ideas of what to eat, there are plenty of anti-inflammatory diet recipe books available.

What Else Can You Do to Reduce Inflammation?

- Chiropractic care boosts immune system and reduces inflammation!

- Reduce exposure to environmental toxins (such as smoke)

- Reduce stress (5)

- Certain types of exercise reduce inflammation - specifically, long term, gradually progressive training, avoiding over-exertion (6)

ABOUT THE ANTI-INFLAMMATORY DIET

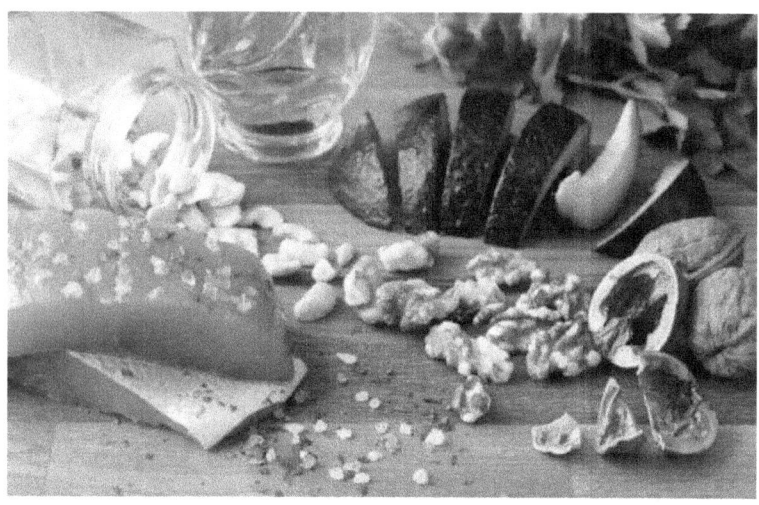

Anti-inflammatory foods are getting tons of hype these days. In fact, just about everyone is using the term "inflammation," from your cardiologist to Tom and Gisele! But keep your baloney detector on.

11   Inflammatory diets are also a thing.

The saturated fat added sugar and sodium in refined carbs and processed snacks make your body's cells work overtime to get their regular job done. Doctors can identify inflammation using biomarkers of oxidative stress, the result of biological processes that cause organ tissue damage. Diet, exercise and smoking status can affect inflammation, but so do uncontrollable causes like autoimmune diseases.

12   It's not just for weight loss.

Anti-inflammatory eating is more of a disease prevention plan. A overwhelming amount of research has shown that people who eat anti-inflammatory foods are at significantly lower risk of developing chronic disease. They're also more likely to maintain healthy weights.

13   Anti-inflammatory foods are everywhere.

The anti-inflammatory diet is often considered a Mediterranean diet, since they recommend the similar foods: Veggies, fruit, whole grains, nuts, seeds, oils, legumes, low-fat dairy and fish. The flavonoids in plants are specifically linked to protecting your body's cells from damage. Both produces and lean protein sources like beans and seafood also contain good-for-you polyunsaturated and monounsaturated fats.

14   You may have these hidden signs of inflammation.

You can't feel inflammation but, if you know what symptoms to look for, you can catch it early, before health conditions emerge. Potential inflammatory warning signs include digestive issues, intermittent joint pain, new food sensitivities, belly fat, worsening allergies, brain fog, unexplained fatigue, moodiness, sleep problems, and rashes.

15   It's inclusive, not exclusive.

Traditional diets always talk about what you can't eat, but when it comes to anti-inflammatory diets, more is more. Colorful foods like leafy greens (spinach, kale), cruciferous veggies (broccoli, cauliflower), carotenoids (tomatoes, carrots) and anthocyanins (beets, berries) are all anti-inflammatory staples.

16   You won't feel hungry.

The plant-based powerhouses known as pulses are an excellent way to incorporate antioxidant- and mineral-rich foods into your everyday life. Dry peas, beans, chickpeas and lentils combine lean protein, unsaturated fats and fiber, filling you up without messing with your diet.

17   Wine and coffee are encouraged.

When it comes to decreasing your risk of Alzheimer's, cardiovascular disease and diabetes, light to moderate alcohol intake of any kind can help. Packed with flavonoids and antioxidants, coffee beans not only ward off cognitive decline, but also boost brain function and stimulation of the central nervous system. Just steer clear of sweetened drinks sugary beverages can increase inflammation!

18   Your mood could get a boost.

Women of childbearing age eat 50% less fish than they should, largely due to previous confusion about prenatal effects. The truth is 12 ounces a week can provide a whole host of anti-inflammatory benefits. Plus, the omega-3's in fish have been linked to a lower risk of depression and reduced anxiety symptoms. Some of our favorite picks include tuna, salmon, sardines, anchovies and other white fish.

19   It's filled with flavor.

Turmeric offers powerful anti inflammatory benefits, says Dr. Corey Kirschner, of the Whole Body Cure, an anti-inflammatory diet plan from our partners at Prevention. Supercharge its anti inflammatory effects by combining it with black pepper, which helps to increase the amount of curcumin (the active ingredient in turmeric) your body can absorb. Turmeric is also fat soluble, he says, so you'll increase your absorption by combining it with a healthy fat like olive oil.

20 Cooking oils are a-okay.

Extra-virgin olive oil is filled with polyphenols, antioxidant-compounds linked to maintaining cell integrity and improving blood flow throughout your body. Canola oil, made from rapeseed, is another anti-inflammatory staple.

21 Conscious indulgences are key.

Ultimately, the anti-inflammatory diet emphasizes real foods as close to nature as possible. But since indulgence is a key part of any eating plan, try treating yourself to about 200 calories of chocolate per day. Research says that eating chocolate regularly may also help maintain a normal BMI. Plus, it can help you cut back on other processed treats.

22 You can try a whole body approach.

Prevention's Whole Body Cure includes 60+ anti-inflammatory recipes, along with the detailed advice you need to reverse chronic inflammation — no prescription required.

23 tomato salad

Just one meal or snack or heck, even a weekend full of fried food cannot induce a state of "inflammation." However, an anti-inflammatory diet may help many people lose weight because it's chock-full of nutrient-dense and delicious foods.

An Anti-Inflammatory Diet For Leaky Gut Disease

Leaky gut disease or leaky gut syndrome is a condition that can be caused by antibiotics, infections, parasites, toxins, or poor diet. The significant feature of the condition is alteration or damage to the bowel lining. As the lining becomes more permeable than normal it allows microbes, undigested food, waste, toxins, or large macromolecules to enter. Some researchers believe that these substances have a direct affect on the body; others think the problem is an immune reaction to those substances.

Whatever has caused it for you, you probably just wish the symptoms -- everything from acne and indigestion to anxiety and fatigue to joint pain and constipation, to name a few - would go away. Unfortunately, that wish can lead to treating just the symptoms. If you have Leaky Gut Disease, however, it's important that you don't just address the symptoms. You need to focus on the root causes of the condition.

One -- if not the main one -- of these root causes is diet. While practitioners disagree on a lot of things about Leaky Gut Disease (whether it even really exists, for example), the diet primarily recommended for those suffering from it - the anti-inflammatory diet - is generally acknowledged to be a healthy one for almost everyone.

The anti-inflammatory diet isn't really a diet; it's more of an eating plan. And if you do a little research, you'll find that there's not just one anti-inflammatory diet; there are several, each with a different spin. For our purposes here, I've tried to present what is a "generic" version. This version does share with the others the concept that continued and out-of-control inflammation leads to illness and that following an eating plan that avoids inflaming the body promotes health and can help prevent disease.

In general an anti-inflammatory diet includes:

Plenty of fruits and vegetables

Plenty of whole grains (e.g., brown rice, bulgur wheat)

Lean protein (e.g., chicken, fish)

Anti-inflammatory spices (e.g., curry, ginger)

Omega-3 fatty acids (such as those found in fish, fish oil supplements, and walnuts)

A reduction in

Refined carbohydrates (e,g., pasta, white rice)

Red meat and full-fat dairy foods

Saturated and trans fats

No refined or processed foods

Many who endorse this diet also urge that you avoid refined sugar and products that contain it as well as caffeine and alcohol. And while drugs don't really fall into the diet category, have your doctor review your prescriptions and monitor your own use of OTC drugs, especially NSAIDS.

One word of caution regarding this plan: The effects you experience (i.e., an improvement in your symptoms) will not be as immediate as they would be if you treated yourself with medications. You probably need to give the anti-inflammatory diet at least two weeks versus the hour or two a medicine might take. On the other side, this diet might have a bonus effect not usually found in medications: weight loss!

HISTORY AND PHYSICAL

Age: Increasing age is positively correlated with elevated levels of several inflammatory molecules. The age-associated increase in inflammatory molecules may be due to mitochondrial dysfunction or free radical accumulation over time and other age-related factors like increase in visceral body fat.

Obesity: Many studies reported that fat tissue is an endocrine organ, secreting multiple adipokines and other inflammatory mediators. Some reports show that body mass index of an individual is proportional to the amount of pro-inflammatory cytokines secreted. Metabolic syndrome typifies this well.

Diet: Diet rich in saturated fat, trans-fats, or refined sugar is associated with higher production of pro-inflammatory molecules, especially in individuals with diabetes or overweight individuals.

Smoking: Cigarette smoking is associated with lowering the production of anti-inflammatory molecules and inducing inflammation.

Low Sex Hormones: Studies show that sex hormones like testosterone and estrogen can suppress the production and secretion of several pro-inflammatory markers and it has been observed that maintaining sex hormone levels reduces the risk of several inflammatory diseases.

Stress and Sleep Disorders: Both physical and emotional stress is associated with inflammatory cytokine release. Stress can also cause sleep disorders. Since individuals with irregular sleep schedules are more likely to have chronic inflammation than consistent sleepers, the sleep disorder is also considered as one of the independent risk factors for chronic inflammation.

What is chronic Inflammation?

To back up for a moment, let me give you a very brief primer on inflammation. It's a complex system in our bodies with an ever-growing list of identified components, but the big picture is that it occurs in two main ways. It can be a self-limited response to an injury or infection, for example if you get a paper-cut or a sprained ankle. You'll notice redness, pain, warmth and swelling in the area. But once all the cells from the inflammatory response have done their job and the injury is healed, that inflammation disappears. That's the kind of inflammation you want to happen.

The other kind of inflammation, called chronic inflammation, is the problematic one. It may occur if the immune system is trying to fend off an infection, like Lyme disease, but isn't having success. Or it may occur if the immune system becomes confused, such as in someone who has antibodies to gluten that also end up attacking other parts of the body that resemble gluten. Inflammation also happens when the immune system senses that something isn't right, such as when LDL cholesterol makes its way into the lining of an artery. White blood cells follow, but instead of fixing the problem, they inadvertently make it worse by making the plaque unstable and more likely to rupture

Symptoms of Chronic Inflammation

Some of the common signs and symptoms that develop during chronic inflammation are listed below.

Body pain

Constant fatigue and insomnia

Depression, anxiety and mood disorders

Gastrointestinal complications like constipation, diarrhea, and acid reflux

Weight gain

Frequent infections

Evaluation

Tests for Chronic Inflammation

Unfortunately, there are no highly effective laboratory measures to assess patients for chronic inflammation and diagnoses are only undertaken when the inflammation occurs in association with another medical condition.

The best test to confirm clinically chronic inflammation is serum protein electrophoresis (SPE) which shows concomitant hypoalbuminemia and polyclonal increase in all gamma globulins (polyclonal gammopathy).

The two blood tests that are inexpensive and good markers of systemic inflammation include high-sensitivity C-reactive protein (hsCRP) and fibrinogen. High levels of hs-

CRP indicate inflammation, but it is not a specific marker for chronic inflammation since it is also elevated in acute inflammation resulting from a recent injury or sickness. The normal serum levels for hsCRP is less than 0.55 mg/L in men and less than 1.0 mg/L in women. The normal levels of fibrinogen are 200 to 300 mg/dl. SAA (Serum Amyloid A) can also mark inflammation but is not a standardized test.

Detecting pro-inflammatory cytokines like tumor necrosis factor-alpha (TNF-alpha), interleukin-1 beta (IL-1beta), interleukin-6 (IL-6), and interleukin-8 (IL-8) is an expensive method but may identify specific factors causing chronic inflammation. Again, the assays are not standardized like hs-CRP, fibrinogen, and SPE.

Treatment / Management

Many dietary and lifestyle changes may be helpful in removing inflammation triggers and reducing chronic inflammation as listed below. The most effective is weight loss.

Low-glycemic diet: Diet with a high glycemic index is related to high risk of stroke, coronary heart disease, and type 2 diabetes mellitus. It is beneficial to limit consumption of inflammation-promoting foods like sodas, refined carbohydrates, fructose corn syrup in a diet.

Reduce intake of total, saturated fat and trans fats: Some dietary saturated and synthetic trans-fats aggravate inflammation, while omega-3 polyunsaturated fats appear to be anti-inflammatory. Processed and packaged foods that contain trans fats such as processed seed and vegetable oils, baked goods (like soybean and corn oil) should be reduced from the diet.

Fruits and vegetables: Blueberries, apples, Brussels sprouts, cabbage, broccoli, and cauliflower, that are high in natural antioxidants and polyphenols and other anti-inflammatory compounds, may protect against inflammation.

Fiber: High intake of dietary soluble and insoluble fiber is associated with lowering levels of IL-6 and TNF-alpha.

Nuts: such as almonds is associated with lowering risk of cardiovascular disease and diabetes.

Green and black tea polyphenols: Tea polyphenols are associated with a reduction in CRP in human clinical studies.

Curcumin: a constituent of turmeric causes significant patient improvements in several inflammatory diseases especially in animal models.

Fish Oil: The richest source of the omega-3 fatty acids. Higher intake of omega-3 fatty acids is associated with lowering levels of TNF-alpha, CRP, and IL-6.

Mung bean: Rich in flavonoids (particularly vitexin and isovitexin). It is traditional food and herbal medicine known for its anti-inflammatory effects.

Micronutrients: Magnesium, vitamin D, vitamin E, zinc and selenium). Magnesium is listed as one of the most anti-inflammatory dietary factors, and its intake is associated with lowering of hsCRP, IL-6, and TNF-alpha activity. Vitamin D exerts its anti-inflammatory activity by suppressing inflammatory mediators such as prostaglandins and nuclear factor kappa-light-chain-enhancer of activated B cells. Vitamin E, zinc, and selenium act as antioxidants in the body.

Sesame Lignans: Sesame oil consumption reduces the synthesis of prostaglandin, leukotrienes, and thromboxanes and is known for its potential hypotensive activity.

Physical Exercise

In human clinical trials, it is shown that energy expenditure through exercise lowers multiple pro-inflammatory molecules and cytokines independently of weight loss.

Conventional Drugs to Combat Chronic Inflammation

Metformin is commonly used in the treatment of type II diabetic patients with dyslipidemia and low-grade inflammation. The anti-inflammatory activity of Metformin is evident by reductions in circulating TNF-alpha, IL-1beta, CRP, and fibrinogen in these patients.

Non-steroidal anti-inflammatory drugs (NSAIDs) like naproxen, ibuprofen, and aspirin acts by inhibiting an enzyme cyclooxygenase (COX) that contributes to inflammation and are mostly used to alleviate the pain caused by inflammation in patients with arthritis.

Statins are anti-inflammatory as they reduce multiple circulating and cellular biomediators of inflammation. This pleiotropic effect appears to contribute in part to the reduction in cardiovascular events.

Corticosteroids also prevent several mechanisms involved in inflammation. Glucocorticoids are prescribed for inflammatory conditions including inflammatory arthritis, systemic lupus, sarcoidosis, and asthma.

Herbal supplements like ginger, turmeric, cannabis, hyssop, and Harpagophytum procumbens are shown to have anti-inflammatory properties however one should always consult with a doctor before their use and caution should be taken for using some herbs like hyssop and cannabis.

Differential Diagnosis

It is important to realize that chronic inflammation is not a specific disease but a mechanistic process. The diseases associated with chronic inflammation are multiple and include CVD, diabetes, malignancy, auto-immune disease, chronic hepatic and renal disease, etc. Hence a good history, physical examination, and routine laboratory tests (glucose, creatinine, liver function, rheumatoid factor, complete blood count, antinuclear antibodies) can confirm or rule out most of the differential diagnoses. Also, pertinent imaging studies will be helpful in certain circumstances, e.g., Inflammatory bowel disease or serum protein electrophoresis for polyclonal gammopathy.

Complications

Although chronic inflammation progresses silently, it is the cause of most chronic diseases and presents a major threat to the health and longevity of individuals. Inflammation is considered a major contributor to several diseases.

Cardiovascular diseases: Many clinical studies have shown strong and consistent relationships between markers of inflammation such as hsCRP and cardiovascular disease prediction. Furthermore, Atherosclerosis is a pro-inflammatory state with all the features of chronic low-grade inflammation and leads to increase cardiovascular events such as myocardial infarction, stroke, among others.

Cancer: Chronic low-level inflammation also appears to participate in many types of cancer such as kidney, prostate, ovarian, hepatocellular, pancreatic, colorectal, lung, and mesothelioma.

Diabetes: Immune cells like macrophages infiltrate pancreatic tissues releasing pro-inflammatory molecules in diabetic individuals. Both are circulating and cellular biomarkers underscore that diabetes is a chronic inflammatory disease. Chronic complications linked with diabetes include both microvascular and macrovascular complications. Diabetes not only increases the risk of macrovascular complications like strokes and heart attacks but also the microvascular complications like diabetic retinopathy, neuropathy, and nephropathy.

Rheumatoid arthritis: It is thought to be initiated by an infectious agent or an environmental factor like exposure to cigarette smoke which induces a local inflammatory response in joints, infiltration of immune cells and release of cytokines.

Allergic asthma: A complex, chronic inflammatory disorder associated with inappropriate immune response and inflammation in conducting airways involving a decline in airway function and tissue remodeling.

Chronic obstructive pulmonary disease (COPD): An obstructive lung disease, develops as a chronic inflammatory response to inspired irritants and characterized by long-term breathing problems.

Alzheimer: In older adults, chronic low-level inflammation is linked to cognitive decline and dementia.

Chronic kidney disease (CKD): Low-grade inflammation is a common feature of chronic kidney disease. It can lead to the retention of several pro-inflammatory molecules in the blood and contributes to the progression of CKD and mortality.

Inflammatory Bowel Disease (IBD) is a group of chronic inflammatory disorders of the digestive tract. It can develop as ulcerative colitis causing long-lasting inflammation and ulcers in the lining of large intestine and rectum or Crohn's disease characterized by inflammation of the lining of digestive tract dispersing into affected tissues such as mouth, esophagus, stomach and the anus.

Deterrence and Patient Education

Chronic inflammation can have a deleterious effect on the body and is a key factor causing almost all chronic degenerative diseases. The following are some of the most effective ways to prevent chronic inflammation.

Increase uptake of anti-inflammatory foods: It is important to avoid eating simple sugars, refined carbohydrates, high-glycemic foods, trans fats, and hydrogenated oils. Consuming whole grains, natural foods, plenty of vegetables and fruits such as avocados, cherries, kale, and fatty fish like salmon is helpful in defeating inflammation.

Minimize intake of antibiotics and NSAIDs: Use of antibiotics, antacids, and NSAIDs should be avoided as it could harm the microbiome in the gut causing inflammation in intestinal walls known as leaky gut which in turn releases toxins and triggers chronic, body-wide inflammation.

Exercise regularly to maintain an optimum weight: It is largely known that adipose tissue in obese or overweight individuals induces low-grade systemic inflammation. Regular exercise is helpful not only in controlling weight but also decreasing the risk of cardiovascular diseases and strengthening the heart, muscles, and bones.

Sleep longer: Overnight sleep (ideally at least 7 to 8 hours) helps stimulating human growth hormones and testosterone in the body to rebuild itself.

Stress Less: Chronic psychological stress is linked to greater risk for depression, heart disease and body losing its ability to regulate the inflammatory response and normal defense. Yoga and meditation are helpful in alleviating stress-induced inflammation and its harmful effects on the body.

Features

Most of the features of acute inflammation continue as the inflammation becomes chronic, including expansion of blood vessels (vasodilation), increase in blood flow, capillary permeability and migration of neutrophils into the infected tissue through the capillary wall (diapedesis). However, the composition of the white blood cells changes soon and the macrophages and lymphocytes begin to replace short-lived neutrophils. Thus the hallmarks of chronic inflammation are the infiltration of the primary inflammatory cells such as macrophages, lymphocytes, and plasma cells in the tissue site, producing inflammatory cytokines, growth factors, enzymes and hence contributing to the progression of tissue damage and secondary repair including fibrosis and granuloma formation, etc.

Types of Chronic Inflammation

Nonspecific proliferative: Characterized by the presence of non-specific granulation tissue formed by infiltration of mononuclear cells (lymphocytes, macrophages, plasma cells) and proliferation of fibroblasts, connective tissue, vessels and epithelial cells, for example, an inflammatory polyp-like nasal or cervical polyp and lung abscess.

Granulomatous inflammation: A specific type of chronic inflammation characterized by the presence of distinct nodular lesions or granulomas formed with an aggregation of activated macrophages or its derived cell called epithelioid cells usually surrounded by lymphocytes. The macrophages or epithelioid cells inside the granulomas often coalesce to form Langhans or giant cells such as foreign body, Aschoff, Reed-Sternberg and Tumor giant cells. There are two types:

Granuloma formed due to a foreign body or T-cell mediated immune response is termed as foreign body granuloma, for example, silicosis

Granuloma that are formed from chronic infection is termed as infectious granuloma, for example, tuberculosis and leprosy.

5 SIGNS TO LOOK OUT FOR

If you are striving to keep yourself healthy for now and many years to come, and you want to know what single thing you should be paying attention to more than anything else, it is this: inflammation.

The reason inflammation is so critical is that it has been found to be a player in almost every chronic disease. And if it hasn't been shown to be associated with a chronic disease, it's probably just because no one has looked for it.

You probably wouldn't be surprised to hear that it is a major part of autoimmune diseases since they are all directly caused by the immune system. Maybe you've also already heard that the white cells that sneak into the walls of your arteries are major contributors to cardiovascular disease, meaning it's not just about cholesterol build-up. Perhaps you also know that cancer tends to form in areas that are chronically inflamed. But you might not have expected inflammation to be a component of osteoarthritis, the disease that we doctors thought was just from too much tackle football or tennis (wear and tear of the bones). Inflammation even plays a role in hypertension and depression.

Top 5 Symptoms of Chronic Inflammation

At Parsley Health, one of our main goals is to help people prevent and reverse chronic disease, so we pay a lot of attention to chronic inflammation. We look for symptoms of inflammation beginning at our patients' very first visit. Here are five common indications that someone may have a chronic inflammatory condition:

Body pain, especially in the joints

Skin rashes, such as eczema or psoriasis

Excessive mucus production (ie, always needing to clear your throat or blow your nose)

Low energy, despite sufficient sleep

Poor digestion, including bloating, abdominal pain, constipation and loose stool

We're diving deep into inflammation. Get our newsletter to read every piece as it's published.

The Tests Your Doctor Should Be Doing

Not only do we listen for inflammation in our patients' histories, but we also test for it in every patient we see using these three biomarkers:

White blood cell count

Sedimentation rate (ESR)

High sensitivity c-reactive protein (hsCRP).   (Note: About 1/3 of the adult U.S. population has an elevated CRP.)

Each one of these looks at different components of the blood to see if there is inflammation in the body. They are non-specific, meaning they don't tell us where the inflammation is coming from, but they do clue us in to look harder for it. Taken together, we get a pretty good idea as to whether inflammation is an issue, and we can also use them to track if the inflammation is resolving or worsening.

How to Heal Chronic Inflammation

If all this talk of chronic inflammation and its pervasive effect on chronic disease is getting you nervous, don't worry! You actually don't need to know which cytokine blocks which receptor to know what to do.

Our recommended approach is very similar to what we recommend for health in general:

Remove the foods that are known to cause inflammation, like sugar, dairy and simple carbohydrates.

Avoid foods that you are sensitive to. This is something we often test for or figure out with an elimination diet.

Eat lots of foods that are known to be anti-inflammatory, like leafy greens, colorful veggies, nuts, seeds, herbs and spices (eg, turmeric, ginger and rosemary) and extra virgin olive oil.

Exercise. Regular exercise of moderate intensity improves immune function and decreases inflammation.(Even occasional exercise has benefits, but high-intensity exercise may actually have a detrimental effect on the immune system.)

Minimize stress and optimize how you respond to it.

Supplements such as probiotics, turmeric, resveratrol and fish oil are known to help fight inflammation.

Inflammation is an amazing unifier of most chronic diseases, so if you want to optimize your current and future health, you can do so by minimizing inflammation. Take note if you have symptoms that seem consistent with inflammation, check for it with blood tests, and do your best to adopt an anti-inflammatory lifestyle.

Ways To Reduce Inflammation

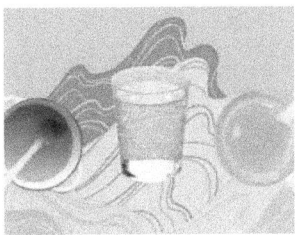

I started connecting the dots between my diet and lifestyle, chronic inflammation, and disease, a light bulb turned on. Why? Because our daily choices are at the root of chronic inflammation.

Over the past decade, I've renovated everything from my grocery cart to my makeup bag to my mind in an effort to upgrade my immune system. And as I moved from a stressful life full of fast food, toxins, and bad boyfriends to a more balanced existence filled with plant-passionate nourishment, inner growth, and conscious living, I started experiencing the perks. Chronic inflammation decreased and my body started working with me to heal and rebuild.

Want to start connecting the dots in your own life? First, let's learn about acute and chronic inflammation, since they play very different roles in our everyday health. Then, we'll cover the causes of chronic inflammation and how to reduce its impact on your health.

The Results of Chronic Inflammation

Over time, chronic inflammation wears out your immune system, leading to chronic diseases and other health issues including cancer, asthma, autoimmune diseases, allergies, irritable bowel syndrome, arthritis, osteoporosis, and even (gasp!) appearing older than your years.

Unfortunately, these challenges are often only treated with drugs and surgery, which may provide temporary relief from the symptoms, but do not treat the root of the problem. In addition, these drugs and their side effects sometimes only add to your health problems.

Could it be that many of the pills in your cabinet are just Band-Aids and that the key to health lies in your daily diet and lifestyle choices? That's certainly what I've found to be true.

The integrative MDs I know and trust are helping their patients identify and address their health issues by looking at the way they lead their lives and nipping their inflammation-happy habits in the bud. If possible, find an integrative doctor who can help you along the way and target your unique needs. They can also test your blood for inflammation make sure your doc requests a CRP—C-reactive Protein test.

Although this may seem overwhelming, it's actually the opposite. The following tips will empower you and help you reduce inflammation over time. Try a few (or just one) of these suggestions on for size and see how you feel. As always, slow and steady wins the race, or in this case, puts out the fire.

How to Reduce Chronic Inflammation

4. Eat more plant-based, whole, nutrient-dense foods.

Crowd out the inflammatory foods we discussed above (refined sugar and flour, processed junk, animal products, etc.) by adding a variety of plant-based whole foods to your diet. These foods will flood your body with the vitamins, minerals, cancer-fighting phytochemicals, antioxidants, and fiber it needs to recover from chronic inflammation.

5. Focus on gut health.

Your gut holds approximately 60 to 70 percent of your immune system, so it stands to reason that it would be a great place to reduce chronic inflammation. And if your gut is in bad shape, you can only imagine that your immune system is in some serious trouble. Check out my tips for improving gut health here. A great way to start is by taking a daily probiotic.

6. Identify and address food allergies and chronic (or hidden) infections.

You could be fighting a losing battle if you're ignoring potential food sensitivities and/or infections. If your body is working to cope and fight these challenges every day, you can bet that you're stoking the fires of inflammation on a regular basis.

Gluten, soy, dairy, eggs, and yeast are common food allergens that might be distracting your immune system every time you sit down for a meal. These allergies can be identified with a blood test. Ask your doctor about testing for food allergies.

Become a symptoms detective. Only you can determine how you feel when you eat, which is where an elimination diet comes in handy. While following the elimination approach, you remove all common allergens from your diet and then slowly reintroduce them, one by one. Talk to your doc about these options, and do some independent research at Google University.

Another possibility worth exploring is chronic infection (bacteria, viruses, yeast, parasites). These guys could be hiding out in your body just under the radar and dragging your immune system down. You have a couple options for testing—look at your bloodwork and/or your poop. It may not be pretty, but knowledge is power, so be brave and have your stool checked. You can have your stool analyzed—this analysis will identify parasites, abnormal bacteria, yeasts, and other gastrointestinal issues, which will help you create a game plan that targets the infection, ideally with the help of an integrative MD or naturopath.

You may also want to look into Leaky Gut Syndrome, a condition that can result in damage to your intestinal lining. When this occurs, bacteria, undigested food, and other toxins can literally leak into your bloodstream, triggering an autoimmune response and a host of painful inflammatory symptoms. A simple urine test can tell you if you need to plug up those leaks, so to speak.

7. Relax and rest more.

Your body is hard at work repairing and restoring your glorious cells while you sleep. Most doctors recommend 7 to 8 hours of sleep per night. If you're cutting corners in the snooze department, you're cheating your immune system, which means it needs to kick into high gear in an effort to keep you well (hello, inflammation).

Stress goes hand in hand with a lack of sleep and a laundry list of demands from daily life. Unfortunately, when you're stressed out all the time, you're also producing more of the hormone cortisol inflammation's BFF. It stands to reason that you can easily reduce chronic inflammation by focusing on stress reduction, whether it's through more sleep, yoga, meditation, long walks, less technology, or a much-needed vacation. You know I love to take every opportunity I can to remind you to take a chill pill.

8. Reduce toxins in your food, home, and personal care products.

Your body's alarm system goes off when you absorb toxic chemicals and pesticides through your digestive tract and your skin. Cut down your exposure by eating organic foods whenever possible and choosing non-toxic personal care and cleaning products.

THE FUNGUS ANTI-INFLAMMATORY DIET AND HOW IT MAY TREAT YOUR NAIL FUNGUS

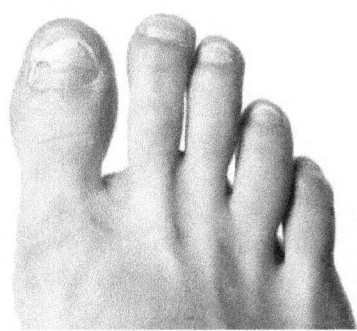

What is nail fungus?

The anti-inflammatory diet can help boost your immune system, which can help fight off fungal infections. Drinking the recommended six to eight glasses of water a day is suggested with this diet, which can help to cleanse your inner system, also helping to fight off infection.

In addition to being helpful in the fight to rid oneself of a fungus infection, there are other health benefits attached to the diet such as help with depression and improved mental state, a stronger immune system, less water retainage and more.

What is the Anti-Inflammatory Diet?

The anti-inflammatory diet usually consists of eating 2,000 to 3,000 calories a day. The amount of calories depends on your size. You should be eating 40 to 50% of carbohydrates, 30 % of fat and include carbohydrates, fat and protein with each meal.

This diet uses a lot of fish and fresh fruits and vegetables while minimizing the consumption of fast food meals. Beans, winter squashes and sweet potatoes are also a big part of this diet.

This diet is not typically meant for weight loss, but can be used for health reasons and is said to help with fungal problems.

How do I know if it's working?

It may take a little while for the diet to work. Remember, if you've been eating a totally different diet, particularly if it was a poor diet, it will take a while for your system to be completely cleaned out. You might want to make a visit to a nutritionist or to the local health food store to discuss how and when the diet will work.

You can expect any treatment to take six to twelve weeks to work and the change in your diet alone may not be enough. Keep a journal of what you eat and do and any changes you see if you are unsure of the effectiveness of treatment.

Okay, I'm on the diet, what else should I be doing?

Again, this is something to be discussed with your healthcare physician, a dietitian or nutritionist or even your health foot store representative who is well-versed in dietary needs. At times, a health foot store may have different or more reliable information than the internet or even your physician's office and may be able to give you some supplements, topical creams or organic lacquers which may prove to be extremely effective, especially in conjunction with the anti-inflammatory diet.

You may also want to check your library or local book store. Internet research can be helpful when making a decision regarding informational books on nail fungus and diet-related and other organic treatment remedies.

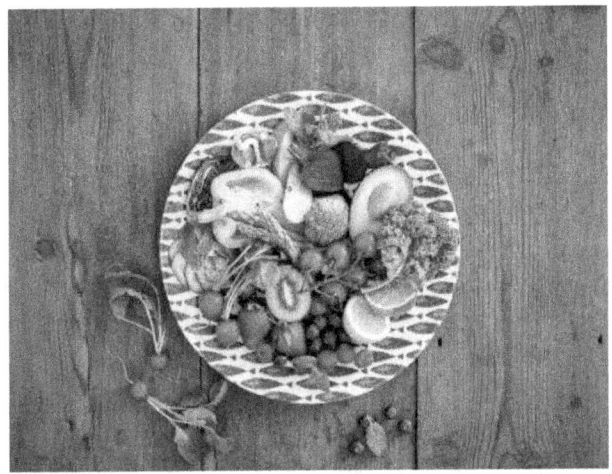

There are a million and one trendy diets out there offering to change how you look and feel in a matter of days. The consumer is flooded with products that will make their skin "appear" healthier and softer to touch. In a world with too much focus on looking good and "appearing" healthier, there is one diet that WILL make you healthier and potentially live a longer life in your anti-aged body.

The anti-inflammatory diet has so many uses today it is surprising every one of the health, fitness and beauty gurus have not jumped on the simplest of diet changes and marketed them as the next big trend in weight loss, beauty and anti-aging. The fact is the anti-inflammatory diet can do everything other diets claim they can do and increase lifespan in the process.

So how do I jump start the anti-inflammatory diet?

Think of this first week as a natural eating time, so don't make any changes or eat anything you would not normally eat. Once the list is complete, head off to the Internet for a little research and education on the power of food over inflammation. Many people are surprised by the effects seemingly healthy foods can have on overall body health and the prevention of illness. Sure, the market screams at the consumer about drinking more vitamin C and reducing calories, but what about the foods that seem healthy but really aren't? These foods will be found after a week of journaling before starting your anti-inflammatory diet.

Are there any baked foods on the list? Chances are, if these foods were purchased prepackaged; they will contain at least a small amount of trans fats. Even the small, 100 calorie bites of cupcake marketed as healthy alternatives can contain up to 0.5 grams of trans fats. Eating just two of these little cakes a day for a week contributes a whopping 7 grams of trans fats - the only healthy level is 0 grams.

Did you eat a salad this week? Many people think eating a salad is a healthy alternative and it can be, without that fat laden dressing covering the healthy greens. One tablespoon of regular dressing can contain 100 calories and about 10 grams of fat. The typical true serving is about ¼ cup per salad. That equates to 400 calories, 40 grams of fat and a -76 rating on the inflammation factor scale which measures the total inflammatory effect of foods on the body.

EATING ANTI-INFLAMMATORY FOODS

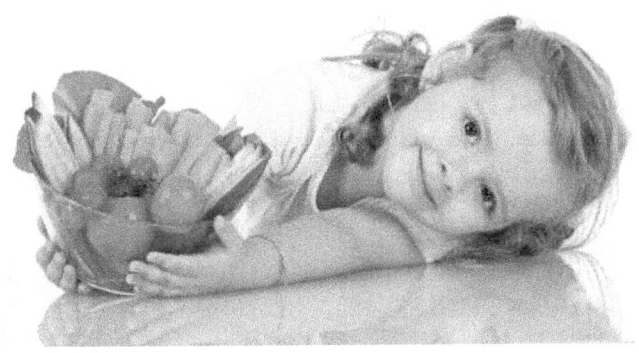

Are there really diets out there that can reduce inflammation? Do they work? Scientists have found that there is a relationship, in part, between what we eat and inflammation. They've even identified some compounds in food that can reduce inflammation and others that promote it. There is still a lot to learn about just how diet and inflammation interact, and research, as of yet, is not at that point where a specific foods or groups of foods can be singled out as being beneficial for people with arthritis. We are beginning to get a clearer picture of how eating the right way can reduce inflammation.

So why are we so concerned about inflammation? Inflammation is the body's natural defense to infections and injuries. When something goes wrong the body's immune system goes to work to inflame the area, which serves to get rid of the invader or to heal the wound. Inflammation can cause pain, swelling, redness, and warmth, but this goes away as soon as the problem is solved. This is good inflammation.

Then we have chronic inflammation, the type that's familiar to people with rheumatoid arthritis (RA), lupus, psoriatic arthritis, and other types of "inflammatory" arthritis.

Chronic inflammation is the type that will not go away. All the types of arthritis that are mentioned above are a disorder of the immune system creates inflammation and then doesn't know when to shut off. Inflammatory arthritis, chronic inflammation can have serious consequences, permanent disability and tissue damage can be one if it isn't treated properly. Inflammation has been linked to a full host of other medical conditions.

Inflammation has been found to contribute to atherosclerosis, which is when fat builds up on the lining of arteries, raising the risk of heart attacks. Also, high levels of inflammation proteins have been found in the blood of people with heart disease. Inflammation has also been linked to obesity, diabetes, asthma, depression, and even Alzheimer disease and cancer. Scientists think that a constant level of inflammation in the body, even if the level is low, can have a number of negative effects. Research shows that diet can reduce inflammation; in theory an inflammation-lowering diet should have an effect on a wide range of health conditions.

Researchers have looked for clues in the eating habits of our early ancestors to discover which foods might benefit us the most. They believe those habits are more in tune to our eating habits with how the body processes and uses what we eat and drink. Our ancestor's diet consisted of wild lean meats (venison or boar) and wild plants (green leafy vegetables, fruits, nuts, and berries). There were no cereal grains until the agriculture revolution (about 10,000 years ago). There was very little dairy, and there were no processed or refined foods. Our diets are usually are high in meat, saturated (or bad) fats, and processed foods, and there is very little exercise. Nearly everything we eat is available close by or as far away as our computer and the click of a mouse.

Our diet and lifestyles are way out of whack with how our bodies are made from the inside out. While our genetic make-up has changed very little from our early beginnings, our diet and lifestyles have changed a great deal and the changes have gotten worse over the last 50 to 100 years. Our genes haven't had a chance to adapt. We aren't giving our bodies the right kind of fuel, it's as though we think of our bodies as engines in a jet plane when instead they are like the engine in the very first planes. There are some foods that we are putting into our bodies, especially because we are eating way too much of them, that are affecting our health in a bad way.

There are two nutrients in our diets that have attracted attention, are omega-3 fatty acids and omega-6 fatty acids have been part of our diets for thousands of years. They are components in just about all of our many cells and are important for normal growth and development. Both of these acids play a role in inflammation. In several studies it was found that certain sources of omega 3's in particular, help to reduce the inflammation process and that omega 6's will raise it.

Now this is the problem, the average American eats on average about 15 times more omega 6's than omega 3's. While our very early ancestor's ate omega 6's and omega 3's in equal ratio, and it is believed that this is what helped to balance their ability to turn inflammation on and off. The imbalance of omega 3's and omega 6's in our diets is believed to contribute to the excess of inflammation in our bodies.

So why is it that we eat so many omega 6's now? Vegetable oils such as corn oil, safflower oil, sunflower oil, cottonseed oil, soybean oil, and the products made from them, such as margarine, are loaded with omega 6's. Even many of the processed snack foods that are so readily available today are full of these oils. Based on the best information of the time, was to use vegetable oils like those mentioned above instead of foods with saturated fats such as butter and lard. It looks like the consequences of that advice may have contributed to the increased consumption of omega 6's and therefore causing an imbalance of omega 3's and omega 6's.

You can find omega 6's in other common foods such as meats and egg yolks. The omega 6 found in meat is the fatty acids that come from grain-fed animals such as cows, lambs, pigs and chickens. Most of the meat sold in America is grain fed unlike their grass-fed cousins who contain less of those fatty acids. Wild game such as venison and boar are lower in omega 6's and fat and higher in omega 3's than the meat that comes from the supermarkets where we shop.

You can get omega 3s in both animal and plant food. Our bodies can convert omega 3s from animal sources into anti-inflammatory compounds more easily than the omega 3s from plant sources. Plant foods contain hundreds of other healthful compounds many of which that are anti-inflammatory, so don't discount them all together.

There are many foods that are high in omega 3s and that include fatty fish, especially fish from cold waters. Of course everyone knows about salmon but did you know that you can also find omega 3s in mackerel, anchovies, sardines, herring, striped bass, and bluefish. It's also widely known that wild fish are better sources of omega 3s than the farm raised ones. You can also buy eggs that have been enriched with omega 3 oils. There are several excellent sources of omega 3s in plants that are leafy greens (like kale, Swiss chard, and spinach) as well as flaxseed, wheat germ, walnuts, and their oils.

You can also get omega 3s in supplements (often as fish oil); this source has been shown to be beneficial in some instances. You should take with your doctor before you take a fish oil supplement because it can interact with some medications and under certain circumstances can increase the risk of bleeding. I take a prescribed omega 3 supplement because my doctor had told me that the ones you get in the supermarket or health food store are not pure, they have other additives that do absolutely nothing to help. There are other fats that are contributors to clogged arteries, the "bad" or saturated fats found in meats and high-fat dairy foods, these are called pro-inflammatory.

There are also the Trans fats that are relatively new to the cause of heart disease. These Trans fats can be found in processed convenience and snack foods and can be spotted by reading the labels. They can be identified as partially hydrogenated oils, often soybean oil or cottonseed oil. But, they can also occur naturally in small amounts in animal foods. The thought is that they contribute to the pro-inflammatory activities in our bodies and the amounts we eat today are staggering.

Antioxidants are substances that prevent inflammation causing "free radicals" from over taking our bodies. Plant foods such as fruits, vegetables (including beans), nuts, and seeds carry high amounts of antioxidants. Extra-virgin olive oil and walnut oil are very good sources of antioxidants, also. These foods have long been considered the basics for good health, and can be found in fruits and vegetables with colorful and vibrant pigments. The more colorful the plant, the better they are for you, from green vegetables, especially leafy ones, to low-starch vegetables, such as broccoli and cauliflower, to berries, tomatoes, and brightly colored orange and yellow fruits and vegetables.

I bet you're wondering what this has to do with Arthritis. Well, there has been some research on diet and arthritis, mostly focusing on RA. There was a study that looked into a bunch of other studies on diet and RA and found that diets high in omega 3's had some effect on reducing the symptoms of RA. There was yet another study published in 2008, that found eating omega 6 fatty acids and omega 3 fatty acids in a ratio of 2 or 3 to 1 (a low ratio compared to the 15 to 1 ratio in most people's diet) decreased the inflammation in people with RA. There was also another study that found taking omega 3 may also allow people to reduce their use of no steroidal anti-inflammatory drugs (NSAIDs), such as ibuprofen (Advil, Motrin) and naproxen (Aleve). But these and other studies don't offer enough evidence to prove that there is any particular anti-inflammatory diet that can have a real impact on arthritis symptoms. It doesn't mean that the diets are harmful; it just means that there may come a day when research may be able to prove their benefits. In the future, diet may be considered one of the many tools along with exercise and medicine that can be used to ease the symptoms of arthritis.

We don't have to revert back completely to the caveman to eat the anti-inflammatory way to benefit from the anti-inflammatory diet. Just eating a healthful diet that is recommended today is right on track. Our chief strategy should be to balance the amount of modern day foods with the foods of long ago, which were rich in the inflammation reducing foods. Really, all we have to do is replace foods rich in omega 6 with foods rich in omega 3, cutting down on how much meat and poultry we eat while eating oily fish a couple of times a week and adding more varieties of colorful fruits and vegetables, and while whole grains were not a part of our early ancestor's diet, it should be included in ours. Be sure that it is whole grains and not refined grains because they contain many beneficial nutrients and inflammation-tempering compounds. Researchers have found that eating a lot of foods high in sugar and white flour may promote inflammation, although there is more studying that needs to be done on the subject.

The amounts of knowledge we have on how the body works and how our ancestor's ate is helping to confirm the old adage: "You are what you eat." But, there is still more we need to learn before we can prescribe any one anti-inflammatory diet. Our genetic makeup and the severity of our health condition will determine the benefits we get from an anti-inflammatory diet and unfortunately there is doubt that there will be one diet that fits us all.

Also, what we eat or don't eat is just a small part of the whole story. We are not as physically active as our ancestors and physical activity has its own anti-inflammatory effects. Our ancestors were also much leaner than we are and body fat is active tissue that can make inflammatory producing compounds.

Anti-inflammatory eating is a way of selecting foods that are more in tune with what the body actually needs. We can achieve a more balanced diet by going back to our roots. If you look at the diet of the people of the Bible, you will find that they, like our caveman ancestors, were more active and their diets consisted of much the same things as our caveman ancestors. They also had no choice but to walk everywhere they wanted to go, there was no such thing as cars or trucks. While we have it easier today, our health has suffered greatly from it.

FOODS THAT FIGHT INFLAMMATION

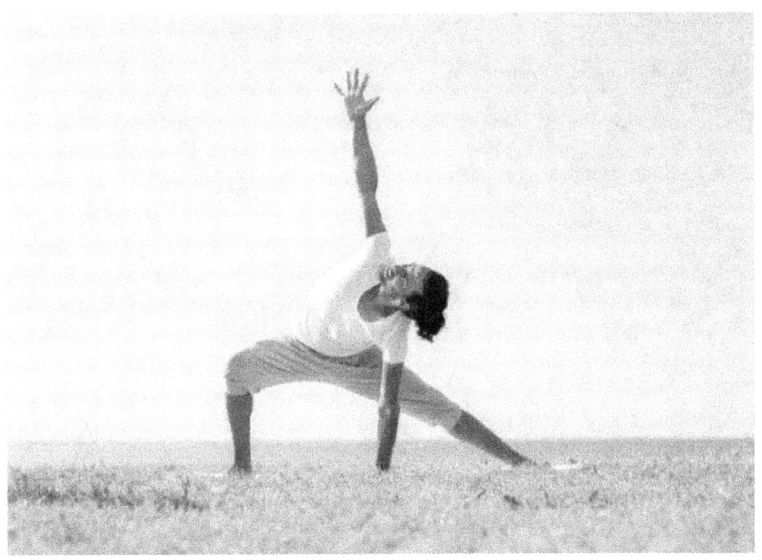

Your immune system becomes activated when your body recognizes anything that is foreign such as an invading microbe, plant pollen, or chemical. This often triggers a process called inflammation. Intermittent bouts of inflammation directed at truly threatening invaders protect your health.

However, sometimes inflammation persists, day in and day out, even when you are not threatened by a foreign invader. That's when inflammation can become your enemy. Many major diseases that plague us including cancer, heart disease, diabetes, arthritis, depression, and Alzheimer's have been linked to chronic inflammation.

Choose the right anti-inflammatory foods, and you may be able to reduce your risk of illness. Consistently pick the wrong ones, and you could accelerate the inflammatory disease process.

Foods that cause inflammation

Try to avoid or limit these foods as much as possible:

refined carbohydrates, such as white bread and pastries

French fries and other fried foods

soda and other sugar-sweetened beverages

red meat (burgers, steaks) and processed meat (hot dogs, sausage)

margarine, shortening, and lard.

The health risks of inflammatory foods

Not surprisingly, the same foods on an inflammation diet are generally considered bad for our health, including sodas and refined carbohydrates, as well as red meat and processed meats.

"Some of the foods that have been associated with an increased risk for chronic diseases such as type 2 diabetes and heart disease are also associated with excess inflammation. "It's not surprising, since inflammation is an important underlying mechanism for the development of these diseases."

Unhealthy foods also contribute to weight gain, which is itself a risk factor for inflammation. Yet in several studies, even after researchers took obesity into account, the link between foods and inflammation remained, which suggests weight gain isn't the sole driver. "Some of the food components or ingredients may have independent effects on inflammation over and above increased caloric intake,

Anti-inflammatory foods

An anti-inflammatory diet should include these foods:

tomatoes

olive oil

green leafy vegetables, such as spinach, kale, and collards

nuts like almonds and walnuts

fatty fish like salmon, mackerel, tuna, and sardines

fruits such as strawberries, blueberries, cherries, and oranges

Benefits of anti-inflammatory foods

On the flip side are beverages and foods that reduce inflammation, and with it, chronic disease, He notes in particular fruits and vegetables such as blueberries, apples, and leafy greens that are high in natural antioxidants and polyphenols—protective compounds found in plants.

Studies have also associated nuts with reduced markers of inflammation and a lower risk of cardiovascular disease and diabetes. Coffee, which contains polyphenols and other anti-inflammatory compounds, may protect against inflammation, as well.

Anti-inflammatory diet

To reduce levels of inflammation, aim for an overall healthy diet. If you're looking for an eating plan that closely follows the tenets of anti-inflammatory eating, consider the Mediterranean diet, which is high in fruits, vegetables, nuts, whole grains, fish, and healthy oils.

In addition to lowering inflammation, a more natural, less processed diet can have noticeable effects on your physical and emotional health

The Benefits of an Anti-Inflammatory Diet

One of the most common problems I address with patients involves the treatment of chronic pain. The day-to-day aches and pains that make life sometimes unbearable. Many people feel that being given drugs for the pain is not the answer, and they seek natural remedies instead.

What Causes Pain

One of the most common causes of pain is chronic inflammation. Inflammation can be described as a condition whereby our tissues become irritated due to injury or infection. The symptoms of inflammation include pain, swelling, red discoloration, heat, stiffness, and/or limited range of motion. There are several conditions that can cause chronic inflammation, including autoimmune conditions like Crohn's disease and rheumatoid arthritis. Chronic inflammation has also been thought to be a contributing factor to conditions like Alzheimer's disease and certain types of heart disease.

Avoid Foods that Cause Inflammation

One of the first things you can do to reduce chronic inflammation is to consider removing foods from your diet that are thought to cause inflammation. The most inflammatory foods are the foods with the highest risk of sensitivity and allergy. The most common food allergies and pro-inflammatory foods are mentioned below.

8. Milk and all dairy products (yogurt, cheese, butter, etc.) not only contain lactose, a sugar many people cannot digest, but a substance called casein. Casein is a protein found in dairy products, and can be pro-inflammatory in many people.

9. Wheat and all wheat products (pasta, bread, cookies, cake, etc.) can be very inflammatory in many people. This is because many people are sensitive to products that contain gluten. If you have not been tested for gluten sensitivity or allergy, try giving up wheat products for 6 to 8 weeks and then reintroducing them. If you feel better off without wheat products and worse on them, this might be a sign of gluten sensitivity. (Please note today that there are many kosher products available on the market that are gluten-free.)

10. Eggs, which can also be found in cakes, sauces, protein powders and many baked goods. Some people are allergic to either the egg whites, the egg yolks, or both. Again, if you have not been tested for food sensitivities, try giving this food up for 6 to 8 weeks and reintroducing it to see if you have a reaction.

11. Meat that is not organic but advertised as corn-fed or vegetarian-fed. If you are looking for kosher organic meat, it does exist, and can be found in some health food stores—try first checking online, or going to your local health food store to find out if they can start carrying it. The reason inorganic meat is pro-inflammatory is because it contains high amounts of a substance called arachidonic acid. Arachidonic acid is a substance found in our cells that initiates something called the PGE2 pathway. This is the process by which a cell undergoes inflammation. Thus, it is believed that too much arachidonic acid in the diet can trigger inflammation.

12. All overly processed foods that contain corn syrup and sugar, like candy bars and soda pops, and processed and cured meats, like hot dogs and sausages.

13. Nightshade vegetables, which include potatoes, tomatoes, and eggplants. These foods contain a substance called solanine, which has been found to cause pain and inflammation in some people.

14. Some people may also be sensitive to citrus fruits like oranges, as well as some tropical fruits like papayas, mangos and pineapples.

What Can I Eat on an Anti-Inflammatory Diet?

5. Try to eat fruits and vegetables that are locally grown, organic and in season. You may want to start looking into buying your produce from local farmers' markets, where produce is often the freshest.

6. Eat meat sparingly, and whenever possible choose meat that is organic. Many companies are now producing organic kosher meats. Lean meats like chicken, turkey and fish are best. Please click here for more information on organic kosher meat.

7. Try to eat cold-water fish and smaller fish. They tend to contain the least amount of mercury and the highest amounts of omega-3 fatty acids, which have anti-inflammatory benefits.

8. Begin to add spices found to decrease inflammation like turmeric. Other spices that decrease inflammation include ginger and rosemary.

9. Begin incorporating whole organic beans and whole grains into your diet. There are many delicious stews and soups with which you can begin to experiment, that use many grains with which you might not be familiar. This include quinoa, brown rice, millet, and unbleached barley, to name a few. Whole grains and beans also offer us a wide variety of nutrients and fiber. Fiber has the added benefit of aiding in healthy digestion. Fiber can also be helpful in lowering cholesterol.

10.　Try to choose oils that are cold pressed, like olive oil. These oils are less processed and, unlike margarine, are not solid at room temperature. They are less inflammatory then the hydrogenated oils, like margarine, and are better for the health of the heart.

While some of these changes may be challenging to incorporate into your diet at first, you will find that they can be quite helpful in reducing inflammation and chronic pain, and can help improve your overall health as well.

KEYS TO REDUCING INFLAMMATION

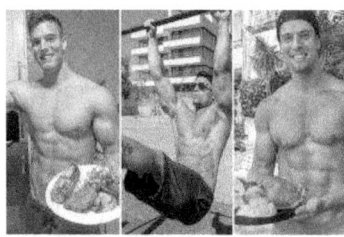

Inflammation (swelling), which is part of the body's natural healing system, helps fight injury and infection. But it doesn't just happen in response to injury and illness.

An inflammatory response can also occur when the immune system goes into action without an injury or infection to fight. Since there's nothing to heal, the immune system cells that normally protect us begin to destroy healthy arteries, organs and joints.

What does chronic inflammation do to the body?

Early symptoms of chronic inflammation may be vague, with subtle signs and symptoms that may go undetected for a long period. You may just feel slightly fatigued, or even normal. As inflammation progresses, however, it begins to damage your arteries, organs and joints. Left unchecked, it can contribute to chronic diseases, such as heart disease, blood vessel disease, diabetes, obesity, cancer, Alzheimer's disease and other conditions.

Immune system cells that cause inflammation contribute to the buildup of fatty deposits in the lining of the heart's arteries. These plaques can eventually rupture, which causes a clot to form that could potentially block an artery. When blockage happens, the result is a heart attack.

What can I do to reduce the risk of chronic inflammation?

You can control and even reverse inflammation through a healthy, anti-inflammatory lifestyle. People with a family history of health problems, such as heart disease or colon cancer, should talk to their physicians about lifestyle changes that support preventing disease by reducing inflammation.

Follow these six tips for reducing inflammation in your body:

5. Load up on anti-inflammatory foods

Your food choices are just as important as the medications and supplements you may be taking for overall health since they can protect against inflammation. "An anti-inflammatory diet emphasizes foods that reduce inflammation.

Eat more fruits and vegetables and foods containing omega-3 fatty acids. Some of the best sources of omega-3s are cold water fish, such as salmon and tuna, and tofu, walnuts, flax seeds and soybeans.

Other anti-inflammatory foods include grapes, celery, blueberries, garlic, olive oil, tea and some spices (ginger, rosemary and turmeric).

The Mediterranean diet is an example of an anti-inflammatory diet. This is due to its focus on fruits, vegetables, fish and whole grains, and limits on unhealthy fats, such as red meat, butter and egg yolks as well as processed and refined sugars and carbs.

6. Cut back or eliminate inflammatory foods

Inflammatory foods include red meat and anything with trans fats, such as margarine, corn oil, deep fried foods and most processed foods.

7. Control blood sugar

Limit or avoid simple carbohydrates, such as white flour, white rice, refined sugar and anything with high fructose corn syrup.

One easy rule to follow is to avoid white foods, such as white bread, rice and pasta, as well as foods made with white sugar and flour. Build meals around lean proteins and whole foods high in fiber, such as vegetables, fruits and whole grains, such as brown rice and whole wheat bread. Check the labels and make sure that "whole wheat" or another whole grain is the first ingredient.

8. Make time to exercise

Make time for 30 to 45 minutes of aerobic exercise and 10 to 25 minutes of weight or resistance training at least four to five times per week.

9. Lose weight

People who are overweight have more inflammation. Losing weight may decrease inflammation.

10. Manage stress

Chronic stress contributes to inflammation. Use meditation, yoga, biofeedback, guided imagery or some other method to manage stress throughout the day.

WHO NEEDS AN ANTI-INFLAMMATORY DIET

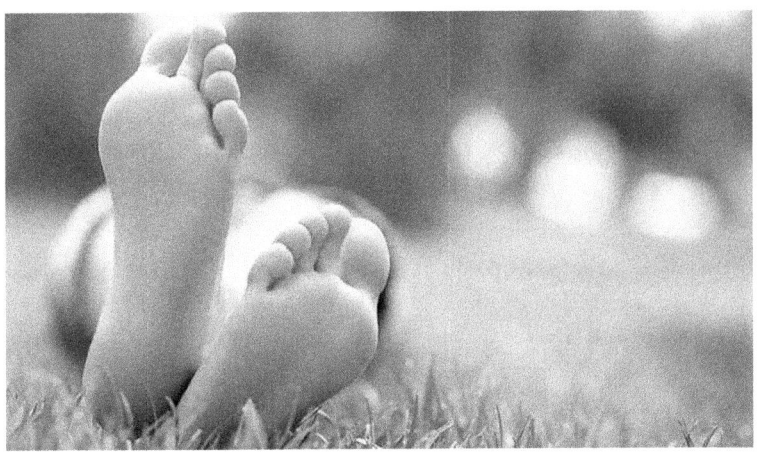

Inflammation is often associated with injury. You stub your toe and the toe swells. This is the basic inflammatory reaction. Some people even understand that redness around a cut is also a form of inflammation that the immune system uses to heal the injury. What is not commonly known is the fact that inflammation occurs inside the body as well. When the body exists in an inflammatory state, risk of illness, cancer and heart conditions can increase. An anti-inflammatory diet is an easy way to combat this aftereffect and reduce risk today.

I Don't Suffer From Inflammation!

This is the most common statement and the least correct. Inflammation affects every person in the world at some point in their life. In western cultures, like the United States, a huge portion of the population is affected by inflammation every day. Being overweight or obese is the most common inflammatory condition. It is this inflammatory response that could be the cause of some weight related conditions like diabetes.

When fat cells grow, they take up the free space around the organs. Blood flow can be constricted and the body often feels as though it needs to fight to function normally. When the body feels threatened, inflammation occurs as a natural, healing response. Unfortunately, unlike the small cut that will heal in a few, short days. Obesity takes time to correct and the longer the body lives inflamed, the greater the risk of long term effects.

In the case of obesity, changing the diet by reducing calories will reduce body weight and thus reduce the inflammation in the body. This is the simplest benefit of an anti-inflammatory diet. However, people who are obese or overweight are not the only people who can benefit from an anti-inflammatory diet.

Illness Treatment and Prevention

There are many illnesses and conditions caused by inflammation. These include asthma, arthritis, inflammatory bowel syndrome, pelvic inflammatory disease, endometriosis, diabetes, COPD, Psoriasis, Colitis, and Lupus - just to name a few. All-in-all, there are nearly 40 autoimmune conditions currently accepted by the medical community that are affected by inflammation.

What Can I Do?

The first step is to make dietary changes to reduce food based inflammation. Processed foods, fast foods and prepackaged foods can cause increased inflammation in the body. Replacing these foods with lean meats, whole grains and healthy fats will make a tremendous different in how the body reacts to inflammation. In addition, if weight is a problem, reducing weight while changing to an anti-inflammatory diet can increase the benefits exponentially.

Changing to an anti-inflammatory diet does not have to be in reaction to a disease or illness. Prevention is the best choice and the anti-inflammatory diet can reduce the risk of contracting many of the listed illnesses. When the body feels as though it needs to fight for survival, inflammation occurs, so offering healthy foods that have an inflammatory effect is a great choice for all people including those who are young, healthy and feel they do not need an anti-inflammatory diet.

STRUGGLES OF AN ANTI-INFLAMMATORY DIET

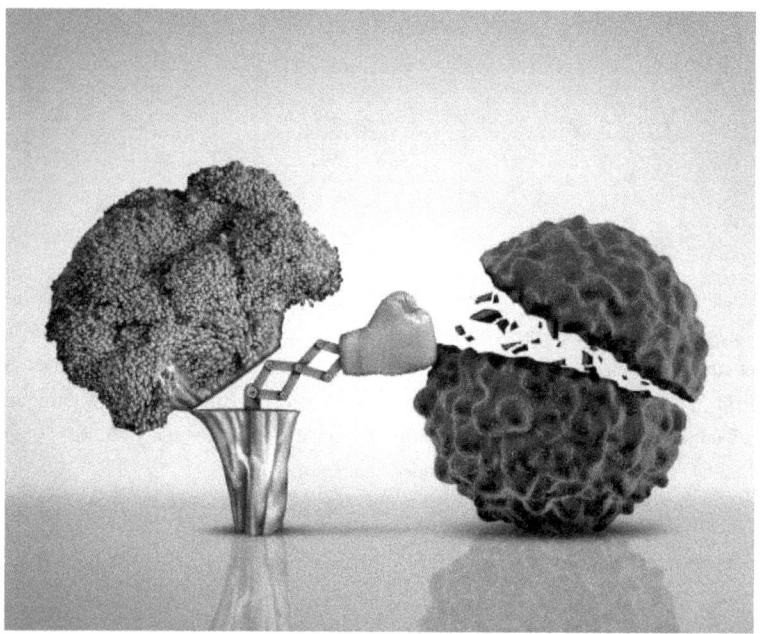

Everyone wants to feel better and live in better health. One of the easiest ways to achieve that is by switching from a traditional western diet to an anti-inflammatory diet. Making the change is easy, but much like a diet plan, sticking with the food changes and watching what you eat can be difficult.

Fast Food and Your Inflammation

Fast food is a huge hindrance to the anti-inflammatory diet. Foods that are high in fat tend to increase inflammatory substances in the body for three to four hours after the meal. If the same number of calories eaten in one fast food sitting were eaten as fresh fruits, vegetables and lean meats, this effect would not occur. Free radicals, cell killers that compound inflammation problems, can also be increased by 175% after eating fast food.

The Alternative - The best alternative to fast food is a replacement, anti-inflammatory diet. This sandwich can be made from lean ground turkey and a whole grain bun. The "special" sauce can be mixed up with lower carbohydrate ketchup, olive oil mayonnaise and sugar free relish. The result is a tasty alternative with a significantly lower fat count.

Red Meat, Milk and Your Inflammation

Science has long fought to connect red meat with certain forms of cancer. Little did they know the research would lead to a link between this common dinner protein and inflammation. Researchers believe the body reacts to certain chemical aspects of red meat and milk in a protective manner. If the body believes these are foreign substances, the immune system will kick in and inflammation occurs. Imagine eating red meat once a day and drinking two or three glasses of milk. The body would live in a state of constant or chronic inflammation which could cause health problems over time.

The Alternative - Lean poultry, beef and fish are all part of a healthy diet. Beef is a great source of iron, so eliminating it is not a necessity. But, choosing the leanest of cuts is essential to good health. The best meats are lean proteins and beans.

Trans Fats and Your Inflammation

A hidden source of body inflammation is the trans fatty acid. While many people know a bit about this type of fat, few understand the effects on the body. Fast food, baked goods, prepackaged meals and margarine are often good sources of trans fat. After entering the body, these fats can increase the risk of coronary artery disease, insulin resistance, diabetes and heart failure. Increased risk of stroke due to abnormally high lipid levels is also common. While many foods will claim to be trans fat free, that is not the entire truth. According to labeling guidelines, these foods can contain up to 0.5 grams of trans fats per serving and still mark the product as "trans fat free". These small amounts will add up over time if the diet is rich in processed foods, margarine and baked goods.

The Alternative - Natural fats like whole butter and olive oil have no trans fats. Choosing these in place of hydrogenated oils and margarine is a good first step. When it comes to foods cooked in trans fat, there is no choice but to eliminate these from the diet all together.

The Anti-Inflammatory Diet for Arthritis Relief

Food and arthritis have a connection to each other and that is why changing your diet is one of the first pieces of advice an expert can give a person with inflammation in his or her joints. There are foods that can reduce inflammation and there are those that might worsen the inflammation. A person with arthritis should follow the anti-inflammatory diet if he or she wants to get treated. To start an anti-inflammatory diet, one should know which foods he or she going to eliminate in one's diet and which foods will be added.

What are the foods that you should avoid and eliminate in your diet? When it comes to arthritis, it is always advised that the person affected should eliminate artificial foods like junk foods, those foods that have been processed and foods with added artificial flavorings and colorings. A person with arthritis should also avoid meats that have high levels of fats and foods that are high in sugar. The reasons why these kinds of foods should be avoided by people with arthritis is that the saturated fats and trans fats found in these kinds of foods can worsen one's condition. He or she should also avoid potatoes, eggplants and tomatoes because these are part of the nightshade family of plant that contains solanine that can provoke the pain. Cutting these kinds of vegetables in people with arthritis have not been proven yet to be effective, but those who followed this kind of diet often show improvements with their condition and find relief from pain.

What are the foods to be added in your diet if you have arthritis? If you already know which kinds of foods you should eliminate in your anti-inflammatory diet, you should now know foods to add to your diet:

1. Healthy fats and Oils: Fish oils are high in Omega-3 fatty acids that are essential to our health. This will help reduce the inflammation and prevent it from coming back. You will also get these fats in some seeds like flaxseed, pumpkin seeds, and sunflower seeds and also in Brazil nuts, almonds, cashew nuts and many more.

2. Fruits and Vegetables: You should be eating more fruits and vegetables if you have arthritis because these have a lot of mineral, vitamins, antioxidants and photochemical that are beneficial for your arthritis and also to other conditions.

3. Protein: Eating more proteins like fishes and other seafoods and poultry meats will also help people with arthritis.

4. Drinks: You should need more liquids to keep your joints lubricated. Drink more water, fruit juices, tea, vegetable juice with low sodium and non-fat milk.

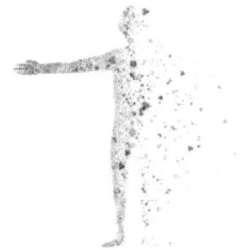

Most people who experience inflammation have heard all about the medications that are available to cure the pain and swelling that can occur during a flare up. But how many know that there are some great anti inflammatory foods that can affect how you feel and reduce the pain associated with inflammation.

Following an anti inflammatory diet will help you beat inflammation naturally.

Inflammation is a swelling that may cause pain, discoloration and even the loss of movement. Usually most people experience severe inflammation when they are the sufferers of arthritis and when they have problems like heart disease and strokes.

Usually your doctor will recommend that you get sleep and exercise in moderation. He may also suggest lowering your weight and taking steroid based drugs or undergoing joint replacement surgery. The medications do work fairly well in reducing the inflammation but often come with some serious side effects, such as ulcers and kidney problems. This may make you wonder if they are worth taking and whether using them is trading one illness for another.

Just like there are some foods that decrease inflammation, there are some that will increase the likelihood that you will get inflammation. These foods are junk foods, fast foods, sugar, and fatty meats. Processed foods that contain Trans and saturated fats also increase the risk of inflammation. Other large contributors of saturated fats are dairy products and eggs. By simply choosing low fat milk, low fat cheese and leaner cuts of meat, you can lower the risks of inflammation, as well as cut down on the chances of chronic disease and obesity. Other foods that increase inflammation include presweetened cereals and soft drinks.

In addition to these, there are foods that are high in sugar and foods that come from the plants labeled as nightshade type. These add to the risk of discomfort associated with inflammation. Eating whole fruits and vegetables will give you the natural healing factors. However, not all vegetables work that way. Potatoes, eggplant and tomatoes can actually make inflammation worse.

So remember the best foods to have are whole fruits, fresh vegetables, lean meats, low fat milk and cheese, as well as fruit and vegetable juices that contain carrots and celery. These types of foods will reduce inflammation and help you get on with your life without pain. Eating right will help you beat inflammation naturally.

A Key to Eating Well

You are what you eat' implies that certain foods can be good or bad for you. They are bad if they are inflammatory foods and good if they are not. If you are a doctor who treats inflammatory conditions, like neck pain or low back pain, wouldn't you want your patients to eat foods that help to reduce inflammation as oppose to consuming inflammatory foods? But how can you tell?

What patients eat can affect their outcome. As a Baltimore chiropractor I have found that review of the literature not only reveals the answer but provides the perfect guide to eating well. So, this article begins with the premise that eating certain foods can actually make things hurt worse-increases inflammation-while eating other foods can actually help lessen pain and promote faster healing. These are known as anti-inflammatory foods and they are closely related to competing omega fatty acids. Swelling, redness, heat and pain occur when tissue become inflamed. It may be overt, like a sprained ankle, or hidden beneath the skin, like in your stomach.

So, what foods should or shouldn't be consumed and why? An example of inflammatory foods are those high in refined or hydrogenated vegetable oils, like potato chips and many baked goods. Refined oils and trans fats are used by manufacturers to extend the shelf life of their products. They are notorious preservatives. On the another hand, olive oil, avocado oil and grape seed oil are natural and are known to be anti-inflammatory. Salmon is very high on the list of ant-inflammatory foods.

The reason has to do with the competing omega fatty acids. "A healthy diet contains a balance of omega-3 and omega-6 fatty acids. Omega-3 fatty acids help reduce inflammation, and some omega-6 fatty acids tend to promote inflammation. The typical American diet tends to contain 14 - 25 times more omega-6 fatty acids than omega-3 fatty acids," according to an excerpt by the University of Maryland Medical System. Now, red meats, such as a good, juicy steak, are high in omega-6 fatty acids. So, does that make it bad? No! It's extremely good for you. A good steak is loaded with essential amino acids and other nutrients. It's just that the key to improving health and reducing inflammation is to balance the amount of omega-6 (e.g., nuts, eggs, poultry, cream, cheese, butter) against the omega-3 (e.g., salmon, tuna, turkey). The saturated fats contained in omega-6 foods compete with the omega-3 foods for vital digestive enzymes, like seagulls fighting over french fries on the boardwalk.

So here's my advice: Limit fatty animal products like red meats and dairy products. Instead, eat more lean cuts of chicken, turkey and fish. Olive oils and avocado can and should replace unhealthy oils from corn, soybeans, safflower, sunflower and other vegetable oils. Sweets should be limited, including all bakery products like cookies, cakes, pies and breads. We all know that our modern diet of processed and fast foods tends to generate inflammation and other evils, like obesity. To counteract bad eating, give close consideration to the competing omega fatty acids.

Here's a suggestion: Quinoa and avocado salad (SERVES 4)

INGREDIENTS:

1 cup red quinoa

2 avocados, cut up in

pieces A few dried

tomatoes

2 fresh basil leaves

1 green onion

Dressing:

½ cup olive oil

Juice of 2 lemons

1 garlic clove (minced)

Salt

Cayenne (very small amount)

DIRECTIONS:

Rinse quinoa in cold water and drain well

In saucepan, bring 2 cups water and ½ tsp. salt to boil. Add quinoa. Cover and reduce heat to low. Cook until water is absorbed (about 20 minutes).

In a bowl, mix together the ingredients in cooled quinoa. Toss with dressing.

AVOIDING INFLAMMATORY FOODS

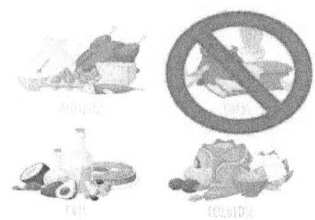

Chronic inflammation continues to threaten the lives of millions worldwide. Today, people are suffering from illnesses such as cardiovascular disease, respiratory disorders, cancers and other inflammatory ailments including familial Mediterranean fever. Developing countries are especially prone to such illnesses and often die from various cancers. Many studies today have shown that lifestyle choices, especially foods we consume everyday, can greatly impact the rate of illnesses.

A well-balanced diet can help fight many of the illnesses people are faced with every day. Some of these foods have anti-inflammatory compounds, which can deter the body from such diseases. As a result, avoiding inflammatory promoting foods and consuming more natural anti-inflammatory foods will greatly reduce the number of illnesses. Here are just a few of the foods that you should avoid which often sets the stage for this inflammatory illnesses.

Alcohol

Found in wines, liquors, and beer, alcohol is often the onset of inflammation in the liver, larynx and esophagus. Chronic inflammation can also develop which promotes tumor growths.

Sugar

Sugar is found in all kinds of candy, desserts, snacks, and beverages. Unfortunately though, excessive amounts of sugar can lead to chronic diseases such as type 2 diabetes, and risk of obesity in addition to inflammatory disorders such as familial Mediterranean fever.

Processed Red Meat

Processed red meat can be found in beef, pork, lamb, salami, and more and should be a red flag. They contain a molecule known as Neu5Gc, which humans do not naturally produce. As a result, ingesting this compound can trigger inflammatory response from the developed anti-Neu5Gc antibodies. These animal products have been known to contribute to colon and rectum cancer in addition to lung and esophagus cancer.

Common Cooking Oils

Cooking oils contain elevated levels of omega-6 fatty acids and low levels of omega-3 fats, not to mention, promotes inflammation and disorders including familial Mediterranean fever. They are used in processed foods and should be avoided at all times.

Artificial Food Additives

Certain food additives are known to trigger inflammation especially in those individuals suffering from conditions like rheumatoid arthritis. These food additives are known as MSG, or monosodium glutamate, and aspartame, which are taste enhancers.

Trans Fats

Trans fats have the tendency of elevated "bad" cholesterol levels while diminishing "good" cholesterol levels, in addition to promoting obesity, insulin resistance and inflammation. They are found in most fast foods, deep fried foods, and commercial baked goods.

Dairy Products

Dairy products are consumed by many people but can not be properly digested. Milk for example, is a common allergen known to induce inflammation and other responses in the intestinal tract. These can all result in constipation, stomach distress, acne, diarrhea, hives, skin rashes, and difficulty breathing.

Refined Grains

Many of the grains consumed today are refined and lack any vitamin B or fiber. They are found in items such as pastries, biscuits, white rice, white bread, white flour, pasta and noodles, and are comparable to refined sugars, however, have an even higher glycemic index, and can trigger degenerative diseases.

Common Inflammatory Arthritis Types

Inflammatory arthritis is arthritis which will inflame the joints. There are many types of this type of arthritis, but to simplify it, I am only going to go over a few types and tell what these types are specifically.

One of the most common inflammatory arthritis types is rheumatoid arthritis. Rheumatoid arthritis can cause a variety of joint pain symptoms as well as other symptoms that make you feel unwell. The symptoms of rheumatoid arthritis are those such as:

1. Intensive joint pains

2. Inflammation of the joints causing swelling

3. Sometimes you may have a rash

4. Fever may be present

Diagnosis of Rheumatoid Arthritis involves something called a SED-RATE blood test. This test will show abnormal results in mostly all people that have rheumatoid arthritis. Another very important test the rheumatologist will certainly do is the blood test which tells the rheumatoid factor in the blood. That factor is always high in the case of people with rheumatoid arthritis.

Upon finding out that Rheumatoid Arthritis is the case, treatments will begin with anti-inflammatory drugs along with a cancer fighting drug called Methotrexate, which my mom has taken for years for rheumatoid arthritis. Methotrexate does wonders for pain reduction of rheumatoid arthritis and helps the person be able to live a happier pain-free life.

Doctors might also use steroid pills or injections to reduce the pain from Rheumatoid Arthritis.

Another inflammatory arthritis type is actually Systemic Lupus. Systemic Lupus is very debilitating over time to the person who has it. The disease brings on symptoms such as:

1. Joint pains, inflammation, and a lot of swelling in the extremo.oInflammatory arthritis is arthritis which will inflame the joints. There are many types of this type of arthritis, but to simplify it, I am only going to go over a few types and tell what these types are specifically.

First, you must understand that any type of inflammatory arthritis is an autoimmune disorder. Autoimmune diseases are those which causes the immune system to launch an attack on its own antibodies, causing various types of medical problems. Inflammatory arthritis is arthritis which will inflame the joints. There are many types of this type of arthritis, but to simplify it, I am only going to go over a few types and tell what these types are specifically.

2. There is definitely skin rashes in many places. 3. Headaches 4. Fevers occur 5. Infections, colds, and flu

Systemic Lupus can be very mild, or very severe. Instead of your immune system creating healthy antibodies, in Systemic Lupus, your immune system prefers to create antibodies that attack major organs.

Treatment for Systemic Lupus involves treating the symptoms that radiate from the disease since there is no cure at this time. Drugs that have an anti-inflammatory effect may help, and a diet that contains foods with properties which help bone and joint pains may ease some of the joint discomfort.

Skin medications and creams may help the various skin type of problems with lupus as well as staying out of the bright sunlight.

Another commonly heard about inflammatory arthritis type is Reiter's Syndrome. Reiter's Syndrome is just as bad as Systemic Lupus in that it causes a lot of joint pain and inflammation, and is very life-limiting as far as being free from pain. This condition is one of those joint diseases that progresses step-by-step, going so far as to affect the eyes conjunctiva, tendons that are latched on to the joints, and the whole body's bone structures, (meaning the skeleton). Interestingly enough, this inflammatory arthritis type comes from sexually transmitted diseases. Venereal diseases carry many types of bacteria strains that cause this dreadful disease.

Symptoms of Reiter's Syndrome are:

1. Genitalia pain since it is coming from bacterias there

2. Multiple joint pains all over the body such as elbows, knees, foot joints, and every possible joint thought of.

3. It is common to have many sores and many rashes

People with Reiter's Syndrome are helped up to a point with anti-inflammatory medications, and possibly Methotrexate, heat therapies for all of the joint pains, and nutritional changes may help.

If the underlying venereal disease is cured or controlled, a lot of the pain from Reiter's Syndrome will clear up since this is the main cause to begin with. To avoid Reiter's Syndrome to begin with, be aware of venereal disease with your sexual partner.

Ankylosing Spondylitis is an inflammatory type of arthritis caused by many years of doing athletics. After a certain number of years as an athlete, bones and ligaments get torn. If this sports related injury is not treated on an ongoing basis, then bone problems will continue progressing until Ankylosing Spondylitis developments within the connective tissues.

This bone issue begins within the sacroiliac joints. This is where both the pelvis and lower spine join together. The symptoms are:

1. Intense back pains

2. Tiredness

3. Trouble with relaxation and breathing very deeply

4. Painful, swollen, red eyes

Treatment for Ankylosing Spondylitis involves getting the immune system back up to where it should be, and the use of steroids and doing blood testing trying to find the reasons for antibodies not functioning properly in the first place. Some of the causes can be due to allergies in foods, and other infectious cycles taking place within the body itself.

FISH OIL'S ROLE IN REDUCING SYMPTOMS OF INFLAMMATORY BOWEL DISEASE (IBD) AND CROHN'S DISEASE

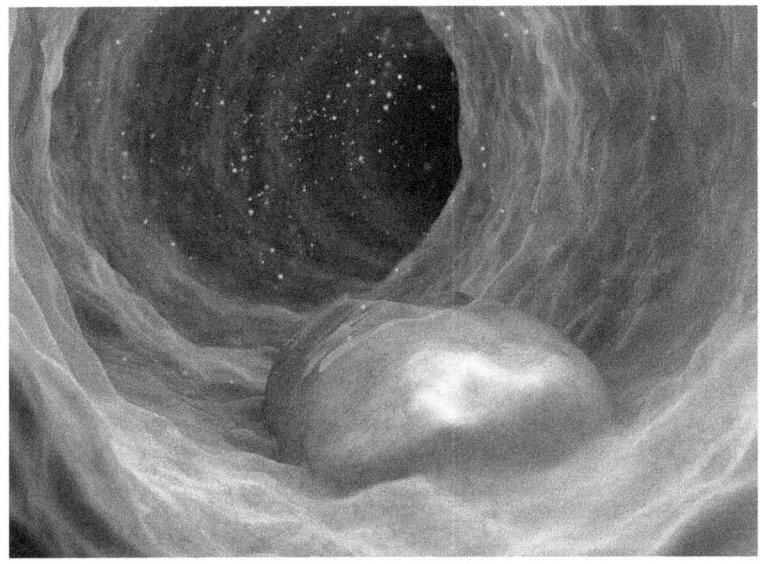

With each passing medical and scientific study the benefits of fish oil and fish oil supplements, are finding their way into the spotlight. Many studies have shown a correlation between reducing the possibility of heart failure, heart attack and different vascular diseases, but it has only been recently that a connection between Omega-3 fatty acids and helpful benefits for patients suffering from Irritable Bowl Diseases (IBDs) such as ulcerative colitis and Chrohn's disease.

Many of these studies are double-blind studies that are further validated with cultural studies of Inuit and Eskimo populations that have a diet high in fish that contains Omega-3 fatty acids and a very low occurrence of ulcerative colitis and Chrohn's disease.

As the evidence mounts, further studies will be needed to pinpoint with any accuracy how much the dietary intake of Omega-3 fatty acids can help in patients suffering from these gastrointestinal diseases, but on the surface the smaller studies that have been done are very promising.

Ulcerative Colitis and Chrohn's Disease Overview

Ulcerative Colitis and Crohn's disease are two types of inflammatory bowel diseases. These diseases are believed to be caused by several factors. First, genetic and non-genetic causes are believed to be the culprit in many cases. The other possible cause is environmental factors such as infections that cause an immune reaction in the gastrointestinal area. The body then generates a large amount of white blood cells in the intestinal lining. These white blood cells release chemicals in the process of fighting the infection that inflame the intestinal tissue. It should be noted, though, that the exact causes of IBDs, such as ulcerative colitis and Crohn's disease, are currently unknown.

In general, an ulcerative colitis attack or Crohn's disease attack will consist of severe intestinal inflammation, which can cause bloody diarrhea, stomach cramps, fever, loss of appetite, weight loss, anemia, bleeding from the ulcers, rupture of the bowel, obstructions and strictures, fistulae, toxic megacolon and malignant cancer. In the last instance, the risk of colon cancer in patients that have had ulcerative colitis or Crohn's disease rises significantly. Generally, after an attack, the disease will go into a remission stage that can last weeks or even years. If you are suffering from these symptoms you should see your physician immediately for a proper diagnosis.

Until recently, the treatment for ulcerative colitis and Crohn's disease was, first and foremost, a healthy diet. If symptoms require it, physicians will ask their patients to limit their intake of dairy and fiber. While it is true that diet has relatively little to no influence on the actual inflammation process within ulcerative colitis, it could have influence on the different symptoms associated with it. On the other hand, diet does have an impact on the inflammatory activity in Crohn's disease and one of the main ways of treating these symptoms is a diet that consists of predigested food. It should also be noted that in both diseases, stress has been shown to be a factor in causing flare-ups. Because of this, physicians will also emphasize the importance of stress management.

Secondarily, medical treatment for these two diseases involves suppression of the high level of inflammatory response mechanisms of the immune system within the intestinal tract. By suppressing this response, the intestinal tissue can heal and the symptoms of abdominal pain and diarrhea can be relieved. After the symptoms have been controlled, further medicinal treatment helps to decrease flare-ups and lengthen or maintain remission periods.

Conventional methods of medicating these two diseases involve a stepped approach. Initially, the least harmful of medications are given in as low a dosage as possible and are taken for a short time period. If these medications provide little or no relief, the dosages are either increased or the medications are changed.

The lowest levels of medications, or Step I, are aminosalicylates and antibiotics. Corticosteroids make up the set of Step II drugs. Step III drugs involve the use of immune modifying medications or a drug called Infliximab for patients suffering from Crohn's disease. These medications are not used, however, during acute flare-ups due to the length of time that a flare-up can last. Only after Step III medications fail completely are Step IV drugs introduced because at this time, they are experimental.

A final alternative in treating ulcerative colitis is surgery. Because ulcerative colitis is limited to the colon, surgery can completely cure it. Crohn's disease, unfortunately, is not restricted to the colon and can exist anywhere in the digestive tract. Because of this, surgery will often complicate matters more.

Limitations of Medical Treatment

Nearly one-quarter of all patients diagnosed with some form of IBD, either Crohn's disease or ulcerative colitis, will not respond to medical treatment. In about three-quarters of cases of Crohn's disease, surgery (even though it is not curative) will be required. Regardless of current medical treatment, a person suffering from ulcerative colitis will have a 50% chance of having remission end within a two-year period after the last flare-up. Even if the initial diagnosis of ulcerative colitis is limited to the rectum there is a 50% probability of the disease becoming more extensive over a twenty-five year period. If a patient has ulcerative colitis that involves the entire colon, that patient stands a 60% chance of requiring a colectomy and most patients will require surgical intervention within the first year after diagnosis of the disease.

It's obvious that Intestinal Bowel Disease can be debilitating. Continued treatments with progressively harsher medications and surgeries that may help in some cases but not others become the norm for these patients. Further, the complications like strictures and fistulas associated with IBDs, can ultimately lead to colon cancer. Many times, these complications create a feeling of hopelessness among those who suffer from ulcerative colitis or Crohn's disease.

There is hope, though. New studies are presenting strong evidence for the use of Omega-3 fatty acids (fish oil and fish oil supplements) in the prevention and treatment of IBDs. These studies are shedding new light on the multi-faceted health benefits of Omega-3 fatty acids and ultimately may present new methods for the treatment of this painful diseases.

The Case for Omega-3 Fatty Acids

Traditionally, the Inuit populations of Alaska have existed on diets high in fatty fish, specifically, types of fish that are high in Omega-3 fatty acids. Past studies of these cultures have shown that the large majority of these groups do not suffer from heart problems, heart disease or other forms of vascular disease. Less known, however, was the fact that the majority of people within these cultures also do not suffer from any form of Inflammatory Bowel Disease. This has led some scientists to postulate that there is a strong connection between the dietary intake of fish oil or fish oil supplements and the prevention of IBDs.

Take, for instance, one example of a symptom of both Crohn's disease and ulcerative colitis: inflammation. Fish oils high in Omega-3 fatty acids have anti-inflammatory properties, which can help reduce its occurrence in patients suffering from IBDs. The reason for this is that when Omega-3 fatty acids are introduced into the body it suppresses the production of leukotriene B4. Omega-3s have also been shown to inhibit interleukin 1Beta. Both leukotriene B4 and interleukin 1Beta are major players in the inflammation of mucosa lining the gastrointestinal tracts.

With regular dietary intake of fish oil supplements high in DHA (docosahexaenoic acid) and EPA (eicosapentaenoic acid), inflammation can be reduced by up to 50% in the intestinal tissues of patients who suffer from ulcerative colitis. Fish oils that have anti-inflammatory properties are only effective in reducing inflammation, but not preventing it. Results in patients with Crohn's disease haven't been quite as promising, but this area of research is still in its infancy.

Recent studies show tremendous promise in fish oil's effectiveness in preventing and reducing the effects of IBDs. These studies show that there is an increase in the manufacture of less powerful prostaglandins at the sacrifice of the more potent ones. Patients with active ulcerative colitis who were given fish oil supplements have also shown significant improvement versus patients who were given placebos. Further study with larger control groups is needed, though, in order for more accurate data to be gathered.

As further evidence of the link between Omega-3s and relief from the symptoms and inflammation of IBDs, a 12-week study involving patients who knew they were taking fish oil supplements showed a significant decline in the disease. This study was further bolstered by the results from samples of the intestinal mucosa that were found to have increased amounts of eicosapentaenoic acid. These results increase when the supplement given to the patients is encased with an enteric coating, which allows the fish oil to be released lower into the intestinal tract. This further alleviates side effects such as fishy breath, burping and flatulence related to taking fish oil supplements. Because of the fewer side effects associated with these supplements, treatment over the long-term is more tolerable.

A Worldwide Phenomenon

With more notice being taken of the effects of Omega-3 fatty acids on the health of people who take them on a consistent basis, the worldwide scientific community has opened up more to the idea of this supplement being used for effective treatment of IBDs. For instance, in Italy, a study was conducted using enteric-coated fish oil supplements and a notable reduction in the rate of relapse in Crohn's disease remission was noted. The patients involved in this study showed evidence of inflammation at the beginning of the study and were suffering from the symptoms related to Crohn's. In this study, patients suffering from the disease received either three fish oil capsules three times per day or a placebo three times per day. Those patients receiving fish oil supplements showed a significant reduction in the inflammation.

Among 39 patients in the placebo group, almost 70% of the patients who were in remission, relapsed. Out of the 39 patients supplementing their diet with fish oil capsules, only 28% relapsed. Further, after a year, nearly 60% of the 39 patients being given fish oil supplements were still in remission while only 25% of the patients given the placebo were in remission.

Given the small size of the study group it is only possible to speculate on the efficacy of treatment for Crohn's disease patients, however, the results of this study are promising. If scientists are given the opportunity to produce a study with a much larger group of patients, better and more accurate data could be gathered which could lead to even more positive results. More research would also allow scientists and doctors to understand the ways in which the EPA works to help increase time of remission.

There is strong speculation that patients suffering from IBDs lack a particular enzyme found in Omega-3 pathways and that when this enzyme is present, remission and even prevention of IBDs is possible. In a sense, adding an Omega-3 supplement to the diet of a patient suffering from Crohn's disease or ulcerative colitis appears to be a type of enzyme replacement therapy.

In Japan, medical researchers at Shiga University of Medical Science conducted a study in which the diet of Crohn's disease patients was altered to include a meal of rice, cooked fish and soup. Prior to the establishment of this diet, the occurrence of relapse within one year was 90%. After implementation of the diet the occurrence of relapse dropped to 40% within one year. Results like this are encouraging other countries to do similar studies.

In the United States, research conducted at Boston University Medical Center shows that patients with chronic IBD have unusual fatty acid profiles that were generally lower than control subjects who did not suffer from any type of chronic intestinal disorder. Because of this lack of fatty acids it is believed that these patients are more prone to these problems. The study also suggests that the addition of Omega-3 fatty acids via a diet that adds fish oil or fish oil supplements can help reduce and correct this shortage.

Another study in San Francisco that involved patients with ulcerative colitis showed that there is an increase in leukotriene B4 in the colonic lining. The hypothesis in this study is that an increase in fish oil supplements in patients suffering from ulcerative colitis could inhibit the synthesis of the leukotrienes. If this is possible, fish oil supplements would be responsible for a reduction or elimination of the symptoms associated with inflammation of the bowels in this disease.

The final results of the study show that the hypothesis was accurate. Patients in the study were randomized and placed into two different groups. The study group received regular daily doses of fish oil containing 2.7 grams of eicosapentaenoic acid and 1.8

grams of docosahexaenoic acid. The second set of patients were placed into a control group and given placebo capsules filled with olive oil. Over a three-month period, patients receiving the fish oil supplements showed marked improvement in the severity of the symptoms of the disease. In fact, 72% of the study group taking the supplements was able to reduce or completely terminate their anti-inflammation and steroid medication schedules.

A similar study done at Mount Sinai School of Medicine shows that the regular use of fish oil supplements in patients suffering from ulcerative colitis diminishes the severity of the disease. Fully 70% of the patients involved in the study showed moderate to significant improvement and 80% of the patients in the study were able to reduce their intake of prednisone, an anti-inflammatory used to help alleviate symptoms of the disease, by up to 66%.

Taking the Next Steps

Studies are showing positive results and it's obvious that the Omega-3 fatty acids inherent to fish oil supplements are beneficial to our intestinal health. The obvious thing to do is find out what types of fish oil supplements are the best. Personal research will aid you in finding the correct supplements and additionally if you suffer from Crohn's disease or ulcerative colitis, you should consult with your physician about the benefits of adding a fish oil supplement to your diet and what dosage you should take. There is, however, some basic information about fish oil supplements that you need to know.

First of all, not all fish oil supplements are created equal. Cod liver oil is, by far, the most inexpensive form of fish oil that contains Omega-3 fatty acids. However, it does not contain the highest amounts and in most cases it cannot be taken in high doses because of impurities such as mercury that are left in it. It also has an extremely powerful taste that most have trouble tolerating.

A much better choice for supplementing your diet with fish oil is a health food grade supplement. These supplements have been purified using a process called molecular distillation. This process eliminates nearly all of the impurities and is very safe when taken in the doses necessary to help alleviate the symptoms associated with IBDs.

The purest form of fish oil supplements is pharmaceutical grade. These supplements have also been processed using molecular distillation, however, at a much higher level. The process used in filtering out the impurities gets rid of all of them down to the particulate level. These supplements, of course, are also the most expensive, but will have the greatest impact on your ulcerative colitis or Crohn's disease.

The benefits of Omega-3 fatty acids are proving to be phenomenal and it is anyone's guess as to the limits of what these supplements can do for our health. With few side effects that are relatively minor, fish oil supplements are a good choice to help you improve your overall health. The fact that they can be used to inhibit the relapse of the symptoms of Crohn's disease and ulcerative colitis is even more exciting. Omega-3 fatty acids are carving out a healthy niche in the diets of individuals worldwide and everyone is all the better for it.

STEPS TO CREATING AN ANTI-INFLAMMATORY DIET

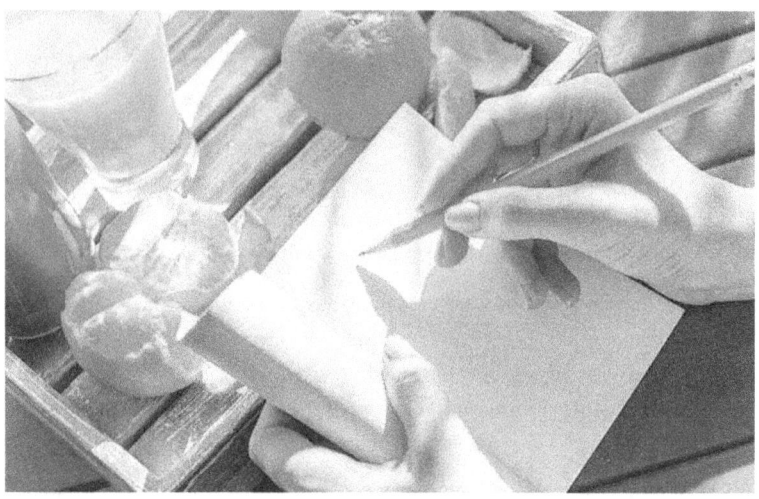

Many diseases such as cancer, cardiovascular disease and autoimmune diseases such as rheumatoid arthritis and celiac disease are linked to chronic inflammation in the body. Luckily, there are many ways to fight inflammation through healthy dietary and lifestyle changes. First and foremost, any dietary modification should begin with a healthy foundation. This includes a balance of lean proteins and healthy fats with a wide variety of colorful fruits, vegetables, grains, and legumes. Variety is the key as focusing on one food, color or nutrient will prevent one from reaping the benefits of all of the others.

There are also many well-known anti-inflammatory foods and nutrients. One of the most researched is omega-3 fatty acids, which are polyunsaturated fats found in foods such as fatty fish like wild salmon, tuna and mackerel, walnuts, chia, flax, and canola oil. A diet rich in antioxidants that includes foods rich in Vitamin C, Vitamin E, and beta-carotene is also known to resist and repair the damage that is induced by inflammation. In addition, phytochemicals in plant foods can also protect against inflammation. Some examples include lycopene, ursolic acid, and lutein. Herbs and spices including turmeric and ginger are also known to have anti-inflammatory properties.

Here are some easy ways to implement an anti-inflammatory diet along with a sample meal plan to help get you started:

Consume a Mediterranean style diet rich in healthy fats such as fish, olive oil, and canola oil; colorful fruits and vegetables; whole grains such as whole wheat pasta and brown rice; and small amounts of lean meats such as skinless poultry breast.

Consume more omega-3 fatty acids from sources such as wild salmon, tuna and mackerel, walnuts, flax, canola oil, omega-fortified eggs. Fish oil supplements that contain both EPA and DHA can be taken under the guidance of your physician.

Consume monounsaturated fat from sources such as avocado, olive oil, and almonds.

Consume more antioxidant-rich fruits and vegetables full of vitamins C, E, and Beta-carotene. Vitamin C can be found in foods such as citrus fruits (oranges, grapefruit), green and red pepper, kiwi, tomatoes, broccoli, and fortified foods. Vitamin E can be found in foods such as wheat germ, vegetable oils, nuts and seeds. Beta-carotene can be found in foods such as carrots, sweet potato, cantaloupe, red pepper, mango, and broccoli

Consume more colorful fruits and vegetables full of phytochemicals such as lycopene, lutein, and ursolic acid. Lycopene can be found in tomatoes, watermelon and red grapefruit. Lutein can be found in dark green leafy vegetables like spinach. Ursolic acid can be found in cranberries, prunes, and apples

Cook with flavorful herbs and spices such as ginger and turmeric. Ginger can be added to soups, stir fry, and homemade tea. Turmeric is used to make curry, casseroles, soups, and stews.

Avoid processed foods, convenience foods, and fast foods which do not contain the healthful properties of an anti-inflammatory diet and contain excessive sodium, preservatives, and saturated fats.

Anti Inflammatory Meal Plan

Breakfast: Add ½ cup berries and ¼ cup shaved almonds to hot or cold cereal

Snack on fruit with low fat or non-fat yogurt or cottage cheese

Lunch: Have a salad with Romaine lettuce, and at least 3 other vegetables that you enjoy (example: carrots, tomatoes, red onions, and cucumber) topped with beans or unsalted plain nuts and olive oil as a dressing

Snack on carrots dipped in hummus

Dinner: Have a stir fry using canola oil including chicken, ground or grated ginger, and red, yellow, and green peppers over brown rice

Snack on a homemade fruit smoothie made with banana, strawberries mixed with skim milk or non-fat yogurt and a tablespoon of ground flax seed.

ANTI-INFLAMMATION DIET FOR DUMMIES CHEAT SHEET

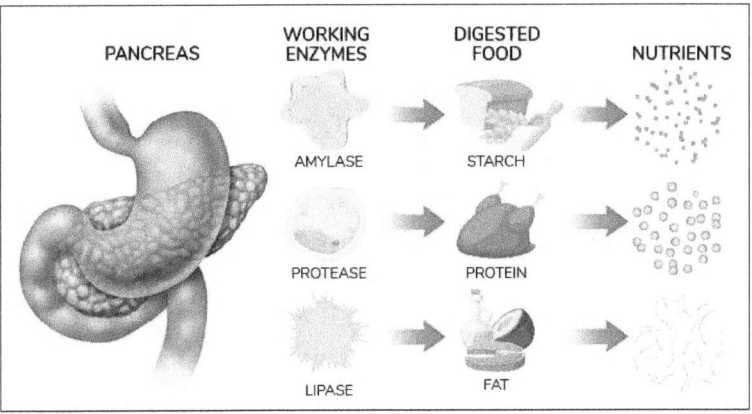

Choosing an anti-inflammation diet is one way to control inflammation in your body. For anyone living with chronic inflammation, finding a way to decrease symptoms and, if possible, erase the inflammation altogether, is a blessing. In many cases, living with inflammation doesn't have to be permanent you can treat, prevent, and sometimes even eradicate those inflammatory issues by knowing which foods are triggers for you, which foods are bad for everyone, and how to change your diet accordingly.

Linking Inflammation to Chronic Diseases

Inflammation contributes to the development and symptoms of chronic illnesses, and understanding that link is the first step in knowing how to change your diet in order to combat inflammation and take better care of yourself. Here are some illnesses linked to inflammation:

Heart disease: Clinical research has linked heart disease from coronary artery disease to congestive heart failure to inflammation. Physicians and researchers provide evidence that the fatty deposits the body uses to repair damage to the arteries are just the start.

Cancer: Foods and proteins, such as fruits and green vegetables, can help you significantly reduce your risks of cancer. Chronic inflammation has been shown to contribute to the growth of tumor cells and other cancer cells.

Arthritis and joint pain: Arthritis has always been linked to inflammation, but it hasn't always been evident that a change in diet could help alleviate the pain and possibly even postpone the onset. Now, however, medical and nutrition professionals see the benefits that natural, vitamin-rich foods can have in relieving the pain of arthritis and possibly even diminishing the inflammation.

Weight gain: It's no secret that food is linked to obesity, but certain foods have a tendency to pile on the pounds more than others. Refined flours and sugars, for example, don't get digested properly and turn to fat much sooner than other, unprocessed foods. Obesity increases inflammation throughout the body by piling pressure on the joints and aiding arthritis, for instance.

Choosing Good Fats for an Anti-Inflammation Diet

Consuming fat in an anti-inflammatory diet isn't forbidden — but the key is knowing which fats are good, which are bad, and which aren't too awful in moderation. "Fat" has become a dirty word in the dietary world, but some fats are not only good for you but necessary for a healthy lifestyle:

Good fats: Polyunsaturated and monounsaturated fats are essential to keeping the good fat in your body in check. Good sources of these fats include olive oil, nuts (almonds, pecans, peanuts, and walnuts, for example), oatmeal, sesame oil and seeds, and soybeans, as well as the omega-3 fatty acids found in salmon, herring, trout, and sardines. The total fat intake for a day should equal between 20 and 35 percent of total calories for the day, and just 10 percent of those calories should be made up of the "bad" fats.

Not-so-good fats: Some foods with saturated fats are okay in moderation, as long as your "moderation" doesn't mean daily. Splurge every now and then, but remember that each splurge takes away from the good you're doing for your body. Sources of saturated fats include fatty meats, butter, cheese, ice cream, and palm oil. Not all saturated fats are bad: Coconut and coconut oil, while considered saturated fats, are actually healthy and beneficial to an anti-inflammatory diet.

Awful fats: Avoid trans fats at all costs. Trans fats are the bad fats found in cakes, pastries, margarine, and shortening, among other foods. One quick and easy way to identify trans fats is to consider the form: Is the fat a solid that can melt and then solidify again? If so, chances are it's a trans fat. Reading the labels on foods is another way to identify trans fats: Hydrogenated or partially hydrogenated fats are trans fats, too.

Making Anti-Inflammatory Food Choices

After you discover the link between inflammation and chronic illness — and the important role food has in fighting them both — you need an idea of what foods will help you treat and even prevent inflammation. Here are some ideas to guide your food choices for different meals:

Breakfasts: Turn to natural ingredients in homemade smoothies, such as berries, honey, and Greek or non-dairy yogurt. Some egg dishes, particularly those made with organic eggs, can help lower inflammation as well. Want toast? Try something gluten- and wheat-free, like rice breads.

Snacks and appetizers: The easiest natural snack is a handful of fruit or fresh veggies. Grab a good crispy apple or a handful of snow peas and you've done your body proud. Want to make it a little snappier? Throw together an avocado dip, stuff an oversized portobello mushroom with kale and other heart-healthy ingredients, or grab a handful of dates. Fruits and nuts are great on-the-go snacks and are filled with vitamins and nutrients, as well as the benefits of omega-3 fatty acids found in most nuts.

Soups and salads: Sometimes there's nothing better than a good cup of soup or a nice salad, but it's easy to get fooled by those that may not be as healthy as they appear. Good soups for fighting inflammation include vegetable soup with a butternut squash base or miso soup with gluten-free noodles. Many people have inflammatory reactions to tomatoes and other nightshade fruits and vegetables, so it's a good idea to stay away from tomato-based soups with potatoes and bell peppers. For salads, steer toward the darker greens and fresh organic toppers, dressed with just a sprinkling of vinegar or olive oil.

Main dishes: Some good anti-inflammatory options for main dishes include most kinds of fish, which is full of omega-3 fatty acids. If you're looking for a bit of protein in your main dish, turn to chicken or even tofu. Try to avoid red meat if possible, but use grass-fed meat if you must go that route.

Desserts: Think "desserts" and the word "sweet" is likely the first to pop into mind — and just because you're trying to fight inflammation doesn't mean you have to fight your sweet tooth, too. Try some chopped fruit and melted dark chocolate to get the vitamins in the fruit and the rich antioxidants in dark chocolate. Need something creamy? Try adding some vanilla extract or honey to a Greek or non-dairy yogurt or, if dairy isn't a problem for you, add it to a little bit of light ricotta cheese.

Changing Your Cooking Methods to Reduce Inflammation

An anti-inflammatory diet begins with choosing the right foods, but it continues with using anti-inflammatory cooking methods to prepare those foods. You can undo a lot of the good in your healthy foods by cooking them the wrong way. Here are some tips on getting the most out of your cooking methods:

Baking: Put your food in the center of a glass or ceramic baking dish, leaving room around the sides to let hot air circulate. Setting veggies on the bottom of a dish, under meat or fish, adds moisture and enhances flavor. Cover the dish to let the food cook with steam while retaining its natural juices.

Steaming: Use a vegetable steamer, rice cooker, or bamboo steamer or create your own steamer with a covered pot and slotted insert to gently cook a variety of foods. Take care, not to overcook vegetables, fish, or seafood. Marinate foods with herbs such as rosemary and sage before steaming, and add spices such as ginger and turmeric to foods while steaming to infuse the flavor into the food.

Poaching: This gentle cooking method requires no additional fats, such as oil. Bring poaching liquid (water or stock, usually) to a boil and add your meat, seafood, or veggies; reduce the heat and simmer until done for a low-fat, flavorful result. Save the poaching liquid from meat or fish and use it as the base of a soup.

Stir-frying: This method allows you to cook with a small amount of oil (or none at all) at high temperatures for a very short amount of time so that the food absorbs very little oil. Vegetables in particular retain their beneficial nutrients.

Grilling and broiling: Reserve grilling for fish and veggies, which don't need much cooking time. Grilling and broiling meats involves excessive temperatures that cause the fats and proteins in meat and protein turn into heterocyclic amines (HAs), which may raise the risk of certain cancers.

Microwaving: As for giving your food a quick zap in the microwave, that convenience appliance destroys the nutrients in food because of the high heat, so you should avoid this cooking method.

RULES FOR OPTIMAL HEALTH OF ANTI-INFLAMMATORY DIETS

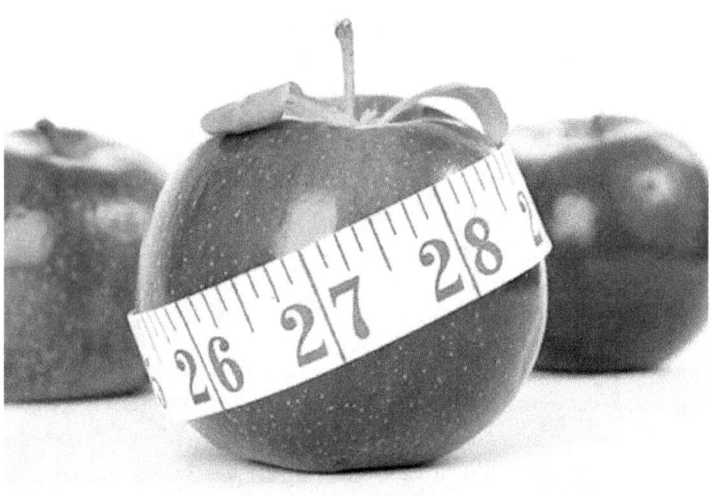

If you want to eat for long-term health, lowering inflammation is crucial. Inflammation in the body causes or contributes to many debilitating, chronic illnesses—including osteoarthritis, rheumatoid arthritis, heart disease, Alzheimer's disease, Parkinson's disease, and even cancer.

Recent research finds that eating this way not only helps protect against certain diseases, but it also slows the aging process by stabilizing blood sugar and increasing metabolism.

Plus, although the goal is to optimize health, many people find they also lose weight by following an anti-inflammatory eating pattern. If you're interested in figuring out what overall diet (Mediterranean, Paleo, etc) is best for inflammation, this is a great article to check out. In general, though, I recommend everyone follow these 11 principles:

1. Consume at least 25 grams of fiber every day.

A fiber-rich diet helps reduce inflammation by supplying naturally occurring anti-inflammatory phytonutrients found in fruits, vegetables, and other whole foods.

To get your fill of fiber, seek out whole grains, fruits, and vegetables. The best sources include whole grains such as barley and oatmeal; vegetables like okra, eggplant, and onions; and a variety of fruits like bananas (3 grams of fiber per banana) and blueberries (3.5 grams of fiber per cup).

2. Eat a minimum of nine servings of fruits and vegetables every day.

One "serving" is half a cup of a cooked fruit or vegetable, or one cup of a raw leafy vegetable.

For an extra punch, add anti-inflammatory herbs and spices — such as turmeric and ginger — to your cooked fruits and vegetables to increase their antioxidant capacity.

3. Eat four servings of both alliums and crucifers every week.

Alliums include garlic, scallions, onions, and leek, while crucifers refer to vegetables such as broccoli, cabbage, cauliflower, mustard greens, and Brussels sprouts.

Because of their powerful antioxidant properties, consuming a weekly average of four servings of each can help lower your risk of cancer.

4. Limit saturated fat to 10 percent of your daily calories.

By keeping saturated fat low (that's about 20 grams per 2,000 calories), you'll help reduce the risk of heart disease.

You should also limit red meat to once per week and marinate it with herbs, spices, and tart, unsweetened fruit juices to reduce the toxic compounds formed during cooking.

5. Consume foods rich in omega-3 fatty acids.

Research shows that omega-3 fatty acids reduce inflammation and may help lower risk of chronic diseases such as heart disease, cancer, and arthritis — conditions that often have a high inflammatory process at their root.

Aim to eat lots of foods high in omega-3 fatty acids like flax meal, walnuts, and beans such as navy, kidney and soy. I also recommend taking a good-quality omega-3 supplement.

And of course, consume cold-water fish such as salmon, oysters, herring, mackerel, trout, sardines, and anchovies. Speaking of which:

6. Eat fish at least three times a week.

Choose both low-fat fish such as sole and flounder, and cold-water fish that contain healthy fats, like the ones mentioned above.

7. Use oils that contain healthy fats.

The body requires fat, but choose the fats that provide you with benefits.

Virgin and extra-virgin olive oil (organic if possible like this one) and expeller-pressed canola are the best bets for anti-inflammatory benefits. Other options include high-oleic, expeller-pressed versions of sunflower and safflower oil.

8. Eat healthy snacks twice a day.

If you're a snacker, aim for fruit, plain or unsweetened Greek-style yogurt (it contains more protein per serving), celery sticks, carrots, or nuts like pistachios, almonds, and walnuts.

9. Avoid processed foods and refined sugars.

This includes any food that contains high-fructose corn syrup or is high in sodium, which contribute to inflammation throughout the body.

Avoid refined sugars whenever possible and artificial sweeteners altogether. The dangers of excess fructose have been widely cited and include increased insulin resistance (which can lead to type-2 diabetes), raised uric acid levels, raised blood pressure, increased risk of fatty liver disease, and more.

10. Cut out trans fats.

In 2006, the FDA required food manufacturers to identify trans fats on nutrition labels, and for good reason — studies show that people who eat foods high in trans fats have higher levels of C-reactive protein, a biomarker for inflammation in the body.

A good rule of thumb is to always read labels and steer clear of products that contain the words "hydrogenated" or "partially hydrogenated oils." Vegetable shortenings, select margarines, crackers, and cookies are just a few examples of foods that might contain trans fats.

11. Sweeten meals with phytonutrient-rich fruits, and flavor foods with spices.

Most fruits and vegetables are loaded with important phytonutrients. In order to naturally sweeten your meals, try adding apples, apricots, berries, and even carrots.

And for flavoring savory meals, go for spices that are known for their anti-inflammatory properties, including cloves, cinnamon, turmeric, rosemary, ginger, sage, and thyme.

MAINSTREAM NUTRITION MYTHS

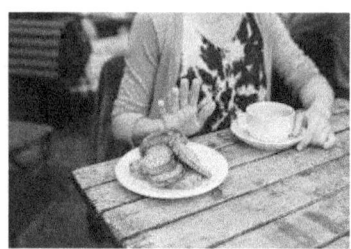

Despite clear advancements in nutrition science, the old myths don't seem to be going anywhere.

Here are 20 mainstream nutrition myths that have been debunked by scientific research.

Myth 1: The Healthiest Diet Is a Low-Fat, High-Carb Diet With Lots of Grains

Several decades ago, the entire population was advised to eat a low-fat, high-carb diet

At the time, not a single study had demonstrated that this diet could actually prevent disease.

Since then, many high quality studies have been done, including the Women's Health Initiative, which is the largest nutrition study in history.

The results were clear... this diet does not cause weight loss, prevent cancer OR reduce the risk of heart disease

Numerous studies have been done on the low-fat, high-carb diet. It has virtually no effect on body weight or disease risk over the long term.

Myth 2: Salt Should Be Restricted in Order to Lower Blood Pressure and Reduce Heart Attacks and Strokes

The salt myth is still alive and kicking, even though there has never been any good scientific support for it.

Although lowering salt can reduce blood pressure by 1-5 mm/Hg on average, it doesn't have any effect on heart attacks, strokes or death.

Of course, if you have a medical condition like salt-sensitive hypertension then you may be an exception.

But the public health advice that everyone should lower their salt intake (and have to eat boring, tasteless food) is not based on evidence.

Despite modestly lowering blood pressure, reducing salt/sodium does not reduce the risk of heart attacks, strokes or death.

Myth 3: It Is Best to Eat Many, Small Meals Throughout the Day to "Stoke the Metabolic Flame"

It is often claimed that people should eat many, small meals throughout the day to keep the metabolism high.

But the studies clearly disagree with this. Eating 2-3 meals per day has the exact same effect on total calories burned as eating 5-6 (or more) smaller meals

Eating frequently may have benefits for some people (like preventing excessive hunger), but it is incorrect that this affects the amount of calories we burn.

There are even studies showing that eating too often can be harmful... a new study came out recently showing that more frequent meals dramatically increased liver and abdominal fat on a high calorie diet.

It is not true that eating many, smaller meals leads to an increase in the amount of calories burned throughout the day. Frequent meals may even increase the accumulation of unhealthy belly and liver fat.

Myth 4: Egg Yolks Should Be Avoided Because They Are High in Cholesterol, Which Drives Heart Disease

We've been advised to cut back on whole eggs because the yolks are high in cholesterol.

However, cholesterol in the diet has remarkably little effect on cholesterol in the blood, at least for the majority of people.

Studies have shown that eggs raise the "good" choleserol and don't raise risk of heart disease

One review of 17 studies with a total of 263,938 participants showed that eating eggs had no effect on the risk of heart disease or stroke in non-diabetic individuals

However... keep in mind that some studies have found an increased heart attack risk in diabetics who eat eggs.

Whole eggs really are among the most nutritious foods on the planet and almost all the nutrients are found in the yolks.

Telling people to throw the yolks away may just be the most ridiculous advice in the history of nutrition.

Despite eggs being high in cholesterol, they do not raise blood cholesterol or increase heart disease risk for the majority of people.

Myth 5: Whole Wheat Is a Health Food and an Essential Part of a "Balanced" Diet"

Wheat has been a part of the diet for a very long time, but it changed due to genetic tampering in the 1960s.

The "new" wheat is significantly less nutritious than the older varieties

Preliminary studies have shown that, compared to older wheat, modern wheat may increase cholesterol levels and inflammatory markers.

It also causes symptoms like pain, bloating, tiredness and reduced quality of life in patients with irritable bowel syndrome.

Whereas some of the older varieties like Einkorn and Kamut may be relatively healthy, modern wheat is not.

Also, let's not forget that the "whole grain" label is a joke... these grains have usually been pulverized into very fine flour, so they have similar metabolic effects as refined grains.

The wheat most people are eating today is unhealthy. It is less nutritious and may increase cholesterol levels and inflammatory markers.

Myth 6: Saturated Fat Raises LDL Cholesterol in the Blood, Increasing Risk of Heart Attacks

For decades, we've been told that saturated fat raises cholesterol and causes heart disease.

In fact, this belief is the cornerstone of modern dietary guidelines.

However... several massive review studies have recently shown that saturated fat is NOT linked to an increased risk of death from heart disease or stroke

The truth is that saturated fats raise HDL (the "good") cholesterol and change the LDL particles from small to Large LDL, which is linked to reduced risk

For most people, eating reasonable amounts of saturated fat is perfectly safe and downright healthy.

Several recent studies have shown that saturated fat consumption does not increase the risk of death from heart disease or stroke.

Myth 7: Coffee Is Unhealthy and Should Be Avoided

Coffee has long been considered unhealthy, mainly because of the caffeine. However, most of the studies actually show that coffee has powerful health benefits.

This may be due to the fact that coffee is the biggest source of antioxidants in the Western diet, outranking both fruits and vegetables.

Coffee drinkers have a much lower risk of depression, type 2 diabetes, Alzheimer's, Parkinson's... and some studies even show that they live longer than people who don't drink coffee.

Despite being perceived as unhealthy, coffee is actually loaded with antioxidants. Numerous studies show that coffee drinkers live longer and have a lower risk of many serious diseases.

Myth 8: Eating Fat Makes You Fat... So If You Want to Lose Weight, You Need to Eat Less Fat

Fat is the stuff that is under our skin, making us look soft and puffy.

Therefore it seems logical that eating fat would give us even more of it.

However, this depends entirely on the context. Diets that are high in fat AND carbs can make you fat, but it's not because of the fat.

In fact, diets that are high in fat (but low in carbs) consistently lead to more weight loss than low-fat diets... even when the low-fat groups restrict calories (35, 36, 37).

The fattening effects of dietary fat depend entirely on the context. A diet that is high in fat but low in carbs leads to more weight loss than a low-fat diet.

Myth 9: A High-Protein Diet Increases Strain on the Kidneys and Raises Your Risk of Kidney Disease

It is often said that dietary protein increases strain on the kidneys and raises the risk of kidney failure.

Although it is true that people with established kidney disease should cut back on protein, this is absolutely not true of otherwise healthy people.

Numerous studies, even in athletes that eat large amounts of protein, show that a high protein intake is perfectly safe

In fact, a higher protein intake lowers blood pressure and helps fight type 2 diabetes... which are two of the main risk factors for kidney failure

Also let's not forget that protein reduces appetite and supports weight loss, but obesity is another strong risk factor for kidney failure

Eating a lot of protein has no adverse effects on kidney function in otherwise healthy people and improves numerous risk factors.

Myth 10: Full-Fat Dairy Products Are High in Saturated Fat and Calories... Raising the Risk of Heart Disease and Obesity

High-fat dairy products are among the richest sources of saturated fat in the diet and very high in calories.

For this reason, we've been told to eat low-fat dairy products instead.

However, the studies do not support this. Eating full-fat dairy product is not linked to increased heart disease and is even associated with a lower risk of obesity.

In countries where cows are grass-fed, eating full-fat dairy is actually associated with up to a 69% lower risk of heart disease

If anything, the main benefits of dairy are due to the fatty components. Therefore, choosing low-fat dairy products is a terrible idea.

Of course... this does not mean that you should go overboard and pour massive amounts of butter in your coffee, but it does imply that reasonable amounts of full-fat dairy from grass-fed cows are both safe and healthy.

Despite being high in saturated fat and calories, studies show that full-fat dairy is linked to a reduced risk of obesity. In countries where cows are grass-fed, full-fat dairy is linked to reduced heart disease.

Myth 11: All Calories Are Created Equal, It Doesn't Matter Which Types of Foods They Are Coming From

It is simply false that "all calories are created equal." Different foods go through different metabolic pathways and have direct effects on fat burning and the hormones and brain centers that regulate appetite

A high protein diet, for example, can increase the metabolic rate by 80 to 100 calories per day and significantly reduce appetite

In one study, such a diet made people automatically eat 441 fewer calories per day. They also lost 11 pounds in 12 weeks, just by adding protein to their diet

There are many more examples of different foods having vastly different effects on hunger, hormones and health. Because a calorie is not a calorie.

Not all calories are created equal, because different foods and macronutrients go through different metabolic pathways. They have varying effects on hunger, hormones and health.

Myth 12: Low-Fat Foods Are Healthy Because They Are Lower in Calories and Saturated Fat

When the low-fat guidelines first came out, the food manufacturers responded with all sorts of low-fat "health foods." The problem is... these foods taste horrible when the fat is removed, so the food manufacturers added a whole bunch of sugar instead.

The truth is, excess sugar is incredibly harmful, while the fat naturally present in food is not.

Processed low-fat foods tend to be very high in sugar, which is very unhealthy compared to the fat that is naturally present in foods.

Myth 13: Red Meat Consumption Raises the Risk of All Sorts of Diseases... Including

Heart Disease, Type 2 Diabetes and Cancer

We are constantly warned about the "dangers" of eating red meat.

It is true that some studies have shown negative effects, but they were usually lumping processed and unprocessed meat together.

The largest studies (one with over 1 million people, the other with over 400 thousand) show that unprocessed red meat is not linked to increased heart disease or type 2 diabetes

Two review studies have also shown that the link to cancer is not as strong as some people would have you believe. The association is weak in men and nonexistent in women

So... don't be afraid of eating meat. Just make sure to eat unprocessed meat and don't overcook it, because eating too much burnt meat may be harmful.

It is a myth that eating unprocessed red meat raises the risk of heart disease and diabetes. The cancer link is also exaggerated, the largest studies find only a weak effect in men and no effect in women.

Myth 14: The Only People Who Should Go Gluten-Free Are Patients With Celiac Disease, About 1% of the Population

It is often claimed that no one benefits from a gluten-free diet except patients with celiac disease. This is the most severe form of gluten intolerance, affecting under 1% of people

But another condition called gluten sensitivity is much more common and may affect about 6-8% of people, although there are no good statistics available yet

Studies have also shown that gluten-free diets can reduce symptoms of irritable bowel syndrome, schizophrenia, autism and epilepsy

However... people should eat foods that are naturally gluten free (like plants and animals), not gluten-free "products." Gluten-free junk food is still junk food.

But keep in mind that the gluten situation is actually quite complicated and there are no clear answers yet. Some new studies suggest that it may be other compounds in wheat that cause some of the digestive problems, not the gluten itself.

Studies have shown that many people can benefit from a gluten-free diet, not just patients with celiac disease.

Myth 15: Losing Weight Is All About Willpower and Eating Less, Exercising More

Weight loss (and gain) is often assumed to be all about willpower and "calories in vs calories out." But this is completely inaccurate.

The human body is a highly complex biological system with many hormones and brain centers that regulate when, what and how much we eat.

It is well known that genetics, hormones and various external factors have a huge impact on body weight

Junk food can also be downright addictive, making people quite literally lose control over their consumption

Although it is still the individual's responsiblity to do something about their weight problem, blaming obesity on some sort of moral failure is unhelpful and inaccurate.

It is a myth that weight gain is caused by some sort of moral failure. Genetics, hormones and all sorts of external factors have a huge effect.

Myth 16: Saturated Fats and Trans Fats Are Similar... They're the "Bad" Fats That We Need to Avoid

The mainstream health organizations often lump saturated and artificial trans fats in the same category... calling them the "bad" fats.

It is true that trans fats are harmful. They are linked to insulin resistance and metabolic problems, drastically raising the risk of heart disease

However, saturated fat is harmless, so it makes absolutely no sense to group the two together.

Interestingly, these same organizations also advise us to eat vegetable oils like soybean and canola oils.

But these oils are actually loaded with unhealthy fats... one study found that 0.56-4.2% of the fatty acids in them are toxic trans fats!

Many mainstream health organizations lump trans fats and saturated fats together, which makes no sense. Trans fats are harmful, saturated fats are not.

Myth 17: Protein Leaches Calcium From the Bones and Raises the Risk of Osteoporosis

It is commonly believed that eating protein raises the acidity of the blood and leaches calcium from the bones, leading to osteoporosis.

Although it is true that a high protein intake increases calcium excretion in the short-term, this effect does not persist in the long-term.

The truth is that a high protein intake is linked to a massively reduced risk of osteoporosis and fractures in old age.

This is one example of where blindly following the conventional nutritional wisdom will have the exact opposite effect of what was intended!

Numerous studies have shown that eating more (not less) protein is linked to a reduced risk of osteoporosis and fractures.

Myth 18: Low-Carb Diets Are Dangerous and Increase Your Risk of Heart Disease

Low-carb diets have been popular for many decades now.

Mainstream nutrition professionals have constantly warned us that these diets will end up clogging our arteries.

However, since the year 2002, over 20 studies have been conducted on the low-carb diet.

Low-carb diets actually cause more weight loss and improve most risk factors for heart disease more than the low-fat diet

Although the tide is slowly turning, many "experts" still claim that such diets are dangerous, then continue to promote the failed low-fat dogma that science has shown to be utterly useless.

Of course, low-carb diets are not for everyone, but it is very clear that they can have major benefits for people with obesity, type 2 diabetes and metabolic syndrome... some of the biggest health problems in the world

Despite having been demonized in the past, many new studies have shown that low-carb diets are much healthier than the low-fat diet still recommended by the mainstream.

Myth 19: Sugar Is Mainly Harmful Because of It Supplies "Empty" Calories"

Pretty much everyone agrees that sugar is unhealthy when consumed in excess.

But many people still believe that it is only bad because it supplies empty calories.

Well... nothing could be farther from the truth.

When consumed in excess, sugar can cause severe metabolic problems

Many experts now believe that sugar may be driving of some of the world's biggest killers... including obesity, heart disease, diabetes and even cancer

Although sugar is fine in small amounts (especially for those who are physically active and metabolically healthy), it can be a complete disaster when consumed in excess.

Myth 20: Refined Seed and Vegetable Oils Like Soybean and Corn Oils Lower Cholesterol and Are Super Healthy

Vegetable oils like soybean and corn oils are high in Omega-6 polyunsaturated fats, which have been shown to lower cholesterol levels.

But it's important to remember that cholesterol is a risk factor for heart disease, not a disease in itself.

Just because something improves a risk factor, it doesn't mean that it will affect hard end points like heart attacks or death... which is what really counts.

The truth is that several studies have shown that these oils increase the risk of death, from both heart disease and cancer

Even though these oils have been shown to cause heart disease and kill people, the mainstream health organizations are still telling us to eat them.

BIGGEST MISTAKES YOU'RE MAKING ON AN ANTI-INFLAMMATORY DIET

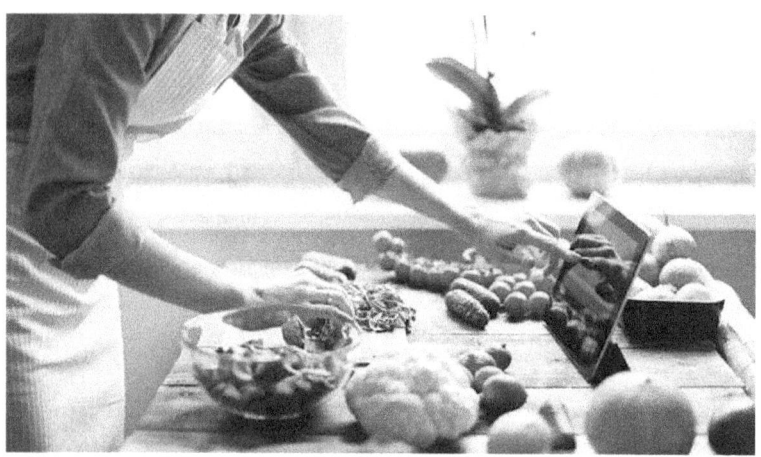

REDUCING CHRONIC INFLAMMATION in the body by way of eating delicious, nutrient-dense foods sound like a dream, but the benefits are as real as it gets.

Inflammation is a healthy response by your immune system that helps your body heal from injury and fights off pathogens like viruses and bacteria. Inflammation becomes harmful when your immune system is triggered into a state of chronic inflammation that runs rampant in your body. In fact, chronic inflammation is at the root of most chronic health conditions and, food is one of the most common triggers of inflammation.

As a nutritionist with an anti-inflammatory approach, I work with clients to help them reduce chronic inflammation in the body. If you're wondering what inflammation is and why you might want to try an anti-inflammatory diet, here is some helpful information.

Is There A Food-Inflammation Connection?

To understand the food-inflammation connection, we look to the gut which has proteins called tight junctions that bind the cells of your gut wall together so that food particles and other substances don't leak through. When you eat food that damages your gut lining, those tight junctions open and enable food particles and other substances to leak through, causing intestinal permeability or leaky gut. This is a problem because the immune cells located just beneath your gut wall identify the food particles as harmful foreign invaders and begin reacting to them. As a consequence, you're left with chronic inflammation, food sensitivities and many resulting symptoms.

Food sensitivity symptoms can manifest anywhere from hours to days after you eat a problem food and can include: skin rashes, acne, excess sweating, hives, fatigue, headaches, migraines, gastrointestinal symptoms, mood issues, asthma, weight management issues, bloating, water retention, muscle pain, joint pain, sinus problems and runny nose, among others.

What Are Considered Anti-Inflammatory Foods?

The best way to combat food-induced inflammation is by adopting an anti-inflammatory diet. On an anti-inflammatory diet, you eat real, whole foods and incorporate anti-inflammatory foods, including:

ginger

turmeric

rosemary

wild Alaskan salmon

oregano

green tea

berries

cacao

cinnamon

garlic

extra-virgin olive oil

flax seeds

tart cherry juice

walnuts

olives

vegetables

Now Tell Me About The Elimination Diet...

When starting an anti-inflammatory diet, an elimination diet is considered the gold standard for helping figure out which foods are inflammatory for your particular system. During an elimination diet, you remove foods that are common inflammatory triggers for a large percentage of the population, such as:

gluten

dairy

soy

corn

eggs

sugar

refined vegetable oils

trans fats

artificial foods

processed foods

fried foods

foods cooked at high heat

refined carbs

Then, after eliminating these foods for a set period of time, you begin to reintroduce some of them one by one to test which may be causing food sensitivity symptoms (see below for more specifics). Keep in mind that if you reduce inflammation and support your gut, in three to six months you can retest a food that you initially reacted to. You may find you do not have any symptoms.

How Do I Start The Anti-Inflammatory Diet?

If you're feeling inspired to eat this way, it's important to set yourself up for success. Even if you understand the basics of the anti-inflammatory diet, it's easy to get tripped up when you're trying it in real life. You should feel empowered to successfully implement the anti-inflammatory diet in your life and stick with it long term.

Here are the most common mistakes that people make when starting an anti-inflammatory diet and how to avoid them:

USING THE ELIMINATION DIET PERMANENTLY Sometimes people feel so amazing during an elimination diet they want to skip the testing component and just stay on the elimination diet forever. But the purpose of an elimination diet is to temporarily restrict certain foods so you can identify which of those foods are inflammatory — it's not to permanently restrict healthy foods from your diet that aren't causing food sensitivity symptoms. People also often remain on an elimination diet indefinitely because they don't know what to reintroduce and so they don't test anything at all. To help you figure out what to test and what not to, here's the cheat sheet:

- There are plenty of nutrient-rich foods that you remove on an elimination diet such as eggs, bell peppers, eggplant and tomatoes — but these foods are a great addition to your diet if they don't cause food sensitivity symptoms. Test these foods.

- Foods with no nutritional value like artificial foods, processed foods and refined carbs are best left out of your diet. You don't need to test these foods.

- Although whole food-based, leave gluten-containing grains out of your diet, even if you don't experience food sensitivity symptoms when you eat them. The reason is that gluten can trigger the release of zonulin, a protein that opens up those tight junctions that bind the cells in the lining of your gut, causing leaky gut.

- Most people feel better leaving dairy out of their diet. However, if you'd like to try adding dairy back in, test it. If you're able to consume dairy without experiencing any symptoms, eat it sparingly and make sure that you choose organic, grass-fed sources that are ethically and humanely produced.

You can also try testing soy and corn, but keep this in mind:

- Make sure you choose organic to avoid exposure to genetically modified sources, which have been engineered to be resistant to the highly toxic herbicide glyphosate.

- If you're going to eat soy, choose fermented sources (like natto and tempeh) and steer clear of the processed versions found in packaged foods.

EATING ORGANIC, GLUTEN-FREE, VEGAN-REFINED CARBS When you start an anti-inflammatory diet and look for swaps for the foods you used to eat, it might be tempting to eat lots of organic, gluten-free and vegan refined carbs such as cookies, chips, pretzels and crackers. But labels like "organic" "gluten-free" and "vegan" don't make any food inherently healthy, and foods with these labels can still be and often are inflammatory.

For example, an organic, gluten-free vegan hot dog bun made from refined flour is totally devoid of nutrients and will still trigger inflammation and spike your blood sugar, even if it's organic and made without gluten or dairy. So, when making substitutions, avoid refined carbs and instead aim to choose swaps made from whole food ingredients.

ADOPTING A DIET MENTALITY | If you only plan to stay on an anti-inflammatory diet until you reach a particular goal, like losing five pounds for example, and then revert to how you ate before, you are defeating the whole purpose of eating this way. Ditch the diet mentality and instead look at this anti-inflammatory nutritional approach as one of the most important lifestyle changes you'll ever make to elevate your health long term. Then, to enable yourself to actually stick with it, focus on finding healthy, delicious ingredient and recipe replacements to take the place of the inflammatory foods you used to eat.

NOT HONORING YOU | Don't let overwhelm prevent you from changing your diet. If it feels too daunting to fully adopt an anti-inflammatory diet right now, ask yourself what would be feasible and start there. In other words, pick one change you feel you're ready to make and commit to integrating it in your life. Once it feels sustainable and effortless — whether it's one day, week or month from now — pick another. Then another. Then another. Before you know it, you will have totally transformed the way you eat, and you will have done it at a pace that was right for you.

BELIEVING ANTI-INFLAMMATORY FOODS CANCEL OUT INFLAMMATORY FOODS | Take as much time as you need to transition to an anti-inflammatory diet while keeping in mind that anti-inflammatory foods can't cancel the impact that inflammatory foods have on your body. So, if you're still eating cheeseburgers and French fries for lunch and dinner, that fish oil supplement and sprinkle of flax seeds on your breakfast while a great start won't help you escape food-induced inflammation.

WHOLE30 DIET FOODS

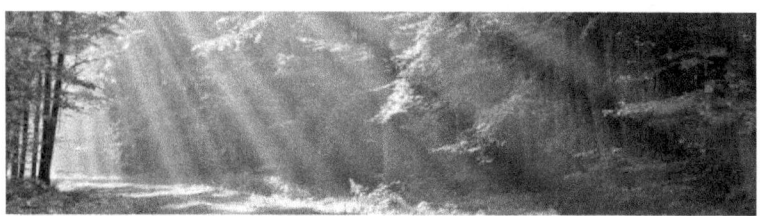

Can Whole30 change your life? We asked an expert to weigh in on this popular eating plan.

Our highly-processed, modern diets trigger inflammation, hormone imbalances, and subtle food intolerances in the body, and the combined effect has a cascading effect on our health, appetite, and cravings. This is the premise behind Whole30, a food "reset" centered around eating only whole, unprocessed or very minimally processed foods.

Struggling to cook healthy? We'll help you prep.

Sign up for our new weekly newsletter, ThePrep, for inspiration and support for all your meal plan struggles.

Focusing on healthy eating changes albeit pretty drastic for most people for a set time period is much more appealing when compared to diets with an infinite end. But how much impact can the Whole30 program really have on health, food cravings, and future food choices? Better yet, is it a safe way to eat long-term? Here's everything you need to know.

What Is Whole30?

By following Whole30 guidelines which include cutting out foods triggering inflammation and imbalances for 30 days you can effectively "calm" your body down. After eating "clean" for 30 days, you can continue with the program or slowly add restricted foods back into your diet. This way, you'll be able to effectively identify which ones may be having subtle effects on your health.

Meals during the 30 day-period center around lots of vegetables, moderate amounts of protein from meat, poultry, seafood, and eggs, some fruits, and healthy fats from foods like nuts, seeds, oils, avocados and olives. Nut milks and nut butters are allowed, as well as all spices and herbs.

Now, here's what you must eliminate or avoid:

All added sugars and artificial sweeteners

Grains (refined and whole)

Legumes, peas, and soy products

Dairy

Highly processed foods and foods with certain additives

Alcohol

While Whole30 isn't usually marketed as low-carb, eating on this plan tends to be lower in carbohydrates. And because some fruits and starchy vegetables like sweet potatoes are encouraged, Whole30 isn't nearly as carb-scarce as the Atkins diet or Keto diet.

In fact, from a macronutrient prospective, a day of Whole30 eating isn't too far off from the current health recommendations (45-65% carbs, 20-35% fat, and 15-25% protein). Here's how a typical Whole30 day breaks down: approximately 35-50% from calories from carbs, 25-35% from fat calories, and 25-35% from protein calories.

What's the Difference Between Whole30 and Paleo?

Whole30 and the Paleo diet both surged in popularity a few years ago around the same time (when their respective books hit the market), and they have lots of similarities. Both diets focus on eating whole, unprocessed foods and cutting out added sugars, grains, legumes, dairy, and processed foods.

However, there are several key differences between the two diets. Whole30 is a strict, 30-day reset period that some then choose to adopt as a long-term eating approach. The Paleo diet, on the other hand, is viewed as a long-term way of living and eating that emphasizes grass-fed, sustainable proteins and local produce. Lastly, nutrient intakes of Paleo followers tend to be a little higher in protein and saturated fat.

Potential Health Benefits of Whole30

While eating according to the Whole30 guidelines may initiate some of these health improvements, this isn't the full picture. These changes aren't necessarily triggered by Whole30 itself but rather the act of following an elimination diet that emphasizes anti-inflammatory eating.

Elimination diets are therapeutic eating protocols that health practitioners have used for years. When a person is plagued by vague, but ongoing symptoms like digestive issues, headaches, joint pain, or skin conditions, they are especially useful in identifying food sensitivities. However, unlike food allergies, food sensitivities are difficult to detect through testing.

Continued consumption of trigger foods can contribute to low-level inflammation and imbalances in the body. Now combines an unknown potential food sensitivity with the typical American diet high in foods that trigger chronic inflammation—added sugars, fried foods, refined carbs, artificial sweeteners, excess alcohol, processed meats, and saturated and trans fats—and you've got a perpetual cycle of inflammation. Research has demonstrated that this type of inflammation increases risks for cancer, type 2 diabetes, heart disease, metabolic syndrome, some autoimmune diseases, and possibly brain alterations.

This is a modal window.

Whole30 is essentially a consumer-friendly version of an elimination diet that cuts out potential food sensitivities for 30 days, as well as drastically decreases inflammatory food intake and increases key anti-inflammatory foods like fruits, vegetables, and omega-3 fatty acids. Whether you have an unidentified food sensitivity or not, the overall effect of eating like this eases inflammation so you could see subtle health improvements related to digestion, skin, headaches, and joint pain.

Potential Problems with Whole30

While the Whole30 diet may be a good "kick-off" for an anti-inflammatory or clean eating approach, its guidelines don't align with research and health recommendations. Among the biggest concerns are the restrictiveness and avoidance of certain food groups. Here are four problems health professionals have when considering this diet as a long-term eating plan:

1. Elimination diets are meant to be temporary.

While extremely helpful to identify foods triggering issues, elimination diets are also very restrictive. They're designed to be a temporary diagnosis tool—and not a permanent way of eating. Elimination diets recommend avoiding certain foods for 4 to 6 weeks, then slowly adding them back one-by-one to identify any triggering issues.

Because Whole30 guidelines don't require the re-entry of restricted foods after 30 days, you may be putting yourself at risk for nutrient deficiencies. Calcium and Vitamin D deficiencies are the biggest concerns, but magnesium, folate, Vitamin A, Vitamin E and others may be affected if you aren't getting an adequate variety of produce and healthy fats.

2. Avoiding Whole Grains.

Consuming whole grains is associated with lowering inflammatory markers in the body and has demonstrated a protective effect when it comes to diabetes and heart disease. The Mediterranean Diet is a key model for anti-inflammatory eating and suggests whole grains be a staple part of one's diet. And unless you're sensitive or allergic to gluten or specific grain, research only supports avoiding refined grains.

3. Avoiding Legumes.

Paleo and Whole30 diets are largely responsible for planting the seeds that beans and legumes should be avoided due to their anti-nutrients. However, these compounds typically have little negative effect on the body—or not nearly enough to outweigh the benefits—when beans are consumed a few times per week. The Mediterranean Diet also recommends legumes as a key source of protein and high-fiber, low-glycemic carbs.

4. Avoiding Dairy.

Unless you have a dairy allergy or sensitivity, there's little research to support avoiding dairy long-term. In fact, dairy products have an anti-inflammatory effect in most people, especially yogurt.

What's the Verdict on Whole30?

The Whole30 diet is a quick snapshot of a healthy, but pretty restrictive, eating pattern. If you frequently consume highly-processed foods and are looking to adopt a healthier lifestyle, you may find the strict parameters helpful. However, research suggests that healthy eating doesn't has to be nearly as limited as the Whole30 guidelines.

ANTI-INFLAMMATORY DIET LIFESTYLE GUIDE

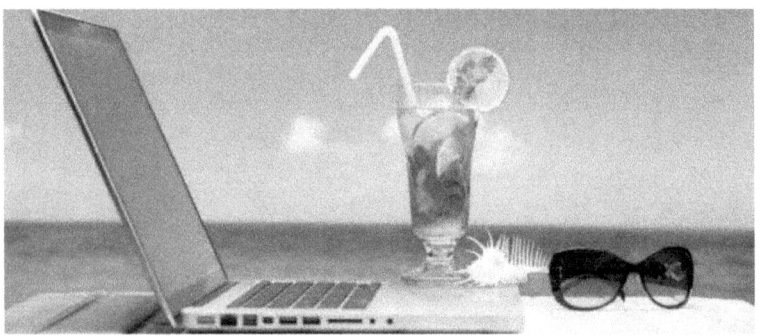

No one among us is utterly immune to inflammation. Even the healthiest people are tripped up at times by a cut on their finger or waylaid by a common cold or flu. Unfortunately, for many of us inflammation is a constant, chronic problem – aches and pains, allergies, autoimmune conditions, cardiovascular disease, diabetes, respiratory issues and more all involve inflammation; it affects millions of people around the world and costs us billions of dollars. The good news is an anti-inflammatory diet and lifestyle can play an important role in the prevention and management of inflammatory symptoms. And it can be delicious!

If you're interested in learning more about how an anti-inflammatory diet can help you, we're sharing our Anti-Inflammatory Diet Guide today. Whether you or someone you love is dealing with inflammation, we hope that you can discover some new ways to address it using our tips and advice.

Dietary changes take time and effort; so don't feel pressured to do everything at once. Incorporate one thing at a time at a pace that feels right to you!

1. Eliminate Sources of Gluten

Gluten, which is found in wheat, barley and rye, is linked to inflammation and can affect the intestinal wall – particles can break through into the bloodstream where they don't belong, leading to an immune response. Gluten has become quite a controversial topic in recent years, with many experts claiming that only those with celiac disease benefit from avoiding and eliminating gluten. However, there are many inflammatory conditions that can benefit from a gluten-free diet, especially those that are autoimmune.

There is no nutrient found in glutenous products that we can't find elsewhere in the diet and in many cases, ditching gluten involves cutting out the junk food like white bread, pizza, pastries, etc. We recommend trying a gluten-free diet for at least two weeks to see how you feel, then adjust accordingly.

2. Ditch the Dairy

Dairy products, especially those made from cow's milk, can be difficult to digest. Many of us don't produce the lactase enzyme required to process the lactose in milk, which can lead to poor digestion and bloating, gas or cramps. Some people react to the proteins in milk like whey and casein and casein is actually similar in structure to gluten.

3. Avoid White, Refined Sugar

It's probably not breaking news to you that refined sugars are damaging to our health. Excess sugar and refined starches spike insulin levels, can boost our body's production of inflammatory chemicals, not to mention that sugar is linked to obesity, diabetes, tooth decay and mood swings.

Thankfully, there are many natural sweeteners available like dates, raw honey, coconut sugar, coconut syrup, maple syrup, etc. And let's not forget about the natural sugars found in fruit, which can be the best dessert of all.

4. Mind The Nightshade Family

The nightshade family includes tomatoes, eggplant, peppers, white potatoes, goji berries and tobacco. Some people are sensitive to nightshade plants, particularly one phytochemical called solanine. Nightshades can impact inflammation, particularly arthritis.

Nightshades can be a tricky food category to navigate, since they also have a multitude of beneficial properties. If you're dealing with inflammation, try cutting them out for a month and see if it makes a difference. You can also rotate nightshades in your diet, as opposed to having them on a daily or weekly basis.

5. Load up on Anti-Inflammatory Foods

The good news is there are a ton – a ton – of delicious anti-inflammatory foods you can include in your diet. These foods are simple to use and easy to find at most grocery stores or farmers markets.

Dark Leafy Greens. These are packed with anti-oxidants that help to ameliorate the effects of inflammation. They also contain a wide variety of other beneficial vitamins and minerals, including B vitamins, iron, magnesium and calcium.

Winter Squash. Winter squash contains curcubitacins, which halt the production of enzymes that lead to inflammation, and they are loaded with immune-supportive Vitamins A and C. Learn more about how awesome they are in this Guide to Winter Squash.

Cruciferous Vegetables. Broccoli, kale, Brussels sprouts, cabbage and cauliflower all help to reduce inflammation and they are a fantastic culinary family to use when detoxing.

Allium Family. Grab onions, garlic, leeks, shallots or chives the next time you're at the grocery store. They contain sulfur compounds and other molecules that avert inflammation; they are also a source of Vitamin C and can help boost the immune system.

Berries. These heavenly fruits are high in a wide range of anti-inflammatory antioxidants.

Fish. Fish is an incredible source of omega-3 fatty acids, which are highly anti-inflammatory, and it's high in protein – an essential macronutrient for healing and repair.

Nuts and Seeds. These are wonderful plant-based option for omega-3s (especially hemp seeds, flax seeds, chia seeds and walnuts). They are also protein-rich and high in fibre.

6. Experiment with Herbs + Spices

There are a range of potent herbs and spices you can add to your pantry that prevent and reduce inflammation, plus they add extra flavour to your meals. Some amazing ones to start off with are ginger, turmeric, fennel, parsley and cumin – but experiment away and see which ones you love to use.

7. Drink Water – And Lots of It

Hydration supports the digestive system, the urinary tract, our joints and our skin; water even helps with energy levels and weight loss. Skip bottled water, which is stored in plastic and is often just tap water. Instead, source the cleanest water you can find, whether that's through buying a water filter or collecting it from a local spring. There are plenty of options out there, and the filters you buy will depend on where you live and what's in your water.

And if you're sick of drinking water plain, here are a few infused water options to jazz things up.

8. Move Your Body

Research indicates that exercise can stimulate anti-inflammatory chemicals in the body and reduce inflammation. Even 20 minutes of exercise like walking is beneficial, so you don't need to run triathlons to reap the benefits. If you're in a lot of pain or are in the midst of a flare up, aim for gentle exercise like walking, swimming, rebounding, hatha or yin yoga, or anything you enjoy at a lighter or more relaxed pace.

9. Lower Stress Levels

Psychological stress can dampen our ability to fight and regulate inflammation. Aim to lower and reduce your stress levels as much as possible; whether it's through yoga and meditation, being out in nature, or eating stress-busting foods, find your stress-reducing sweet spot and live there as much as possible!

It is becoming increasingly clear that chronic inflammation is the root cause of many serious illnesses including heart disease, many cancers, and Alzheimer's disease. We all know inflammation on the surface of the body as local redness, heat, swelling and pain. It is the cornerstone of the body's healing response, bringing more nourishment and more immune activity to a site of injury or infection. But when inflammation persists or serves no purpose, it damages the body and causes illness. Stress, lack of exercise, genetic predisposition, and exposure to toxins (like secondhand tobacco smoke) can all contribute to such chronic inflammation, but dietary choices play a big role as well. Learning how specific foods influence the inflammatory process is the best strategy for containing it and reducing long-term disease risks.

The Anti Inflammatory Food Pyramid Now!

The Anti-Inflammatory Diet is not a diet in the popular sense – it is not intended as a weight-loss program (although people can and do lose weight on it), nor is the Anti-Inflammatory Diet an eating plan to stay on for a limited period of time. Rather, it is way of selecting and preparing anti-inflammatory foods based on scientific knowledge of

how they can help your body maintain optimum health. Along with influencing inflammation, this natural anti-inflammatory diet will provide steady energy and ample vitamins, minerals, essential fatty acids dietary fiber, and protective phytonutrients.

General Anti-Inflammatory Diet Tips:

Aim for variety.

Include as much fresh food as possible.

Minimize your consumption of processed foods and fast food.

Eat an abundance of fruits and vegetables.

Caloric Intake

Most adults need to consume between 2,000 and 3,000 calories a day.

Women and smaller and less active people need fewer calories.

Men and bigger and more active people need more calories.

If you are eating the appropriate number of calories for your level of activity, your weight should not fluctuate greatly.

The distribution of calories you take in should be as follows: 40 to 50 percent from carbohydrates, 30 percent from fat, and 20 to 30 percent from protein.

Try to include carbohydrates, fat, and protein at each meal.

Carbohydrates

On a 2,000-calorie-a-day diet, adult women should consume between 160 to 200 grams of carbohydrates a day.

Adult men should consume between 240 to 300 grams of carbohydrates a day.

The majority of this should be in the form of less-refined, less-processed foods with a low glycemic load.

Reduce your consumption of foods made with wheat flour and sugar, especially bread and most packaged snack foods (including chips and pretzels).

Eat more whole grains such as brown rice and bulgur wheat, in which the grain is intact or in a few large pieces. These are preferable to whole wheat flour products, which have roughly the same glycemic index as white flour products.

Eat more beans, winter squashes, and sweet potatoes.

Cook pasta al dente and eat it in moderation.

Avoid products made with high fructose corn syrup.

Fat

On a 2,000-calorie-a-day diet, 600 calories can come from fat – that is, about 67 grams. This should be in a ratio of 1:2:1 of saturated to monounsaturated to polyunsaturated fat.

Reduce your intake of saturated fat by eating less butter, cream, high-fat cheese, unskinned chicken and fatty meats, and products made with palm kernel oil.

Use extra-virgin olive oil as a main cooking oil. If you want a neutral tasting oil, use expeller-pressed, organic canola oil. Organic, high-oleic, expeller pressed versions of sunflower and safflower oil are also acceptable.

Avoid regular safflower and sunflower oils, corn oil, cottonseed oil, and mixed vegetable

oils.

Strictly avoid margarine, vegetable shortening, and all products listing them as ingredients. Strictly avoid all products made with partially hydrogenated oils of any kind. Include in your diet avocados and nuts, especially walnuts, cashews, almonds, and nut butters made from these nuts.

For omega-3 fatty acids, eat salmon (preferably fresh or frozen wild or canned sockeye), sardines packed in water or olive oil, herring, and black cod (sablefish, butterfish); omega-3 fortified eggs; hemp seeds and flaxseeds (preferably freshly ground); or take a fish oil supplement (look for products that provide both EPA and DHA, in a convenient daily dosage of two to three grams).

Protein

On a 2,000-calorie-a-day diet, your daily intake of protein should be between 80 and 120 grams. Eat less protein if you have liver or kidney problems, allergies, or autoimmune disease.

Decrease your consumption of animal protein except for fish and high quality natural cheese and yogurt.

Eat more vegetable protein, especially from beans in general and soybeans in particular. Become familiar with the range of whole-soy foods available and find ones you like.

Fiber

Try to eat 40 grams of fiber a day. You can achieve this by increasing your consumption of fruit, especially berries, vegetables (especially beans), and whole grains.

Ready-made cereals can be good fiber sources, but read labels to make sure they give you at least 4 and preferably 5 grams of bran per one-ounce serving.

Phytonutrients

To get maximum natural protection against age-related diseases (including cardiovascular disease, cancer, and neurodegenerative disease) as well as against environmental toxicity, eat a variety of fruits, vegetables and mushrooms.

Choose fruits and vegetables from all parts of the color spectrum, especially berries, tomatoes, orange and yellow fruits, and dark leafy greens.

Choose organic produce whenever possible. Learn which conventionally grown crops are most likely to carry pesticide residues and avoid them.

Eat cruciferous (cabbage-family) vegetables regularly.

Include soy foods in your diet.

Drink tea instead of coffee, especially good quality white, green or oolong tea.

If you drink alcohol, use red wine preferentially.

Enjoy plain dark chocolate in moderation (with a minimum cocoa content of 70 percent).

Vitamins and Minerals

The best way to obtain all of your daily vitamins, minerals, and micronutrients is by eating a diet high in fresh foods with an abundance of fruits and vegetables. In addition, supplement your diet with the following antioxidant cocktail:

Vitamin C, 200 milligrams a day.

Vitamin E. Most adults should limit their daily supplement intake of vitamin E to 100-200 IU (in the form of mixed tocopherols and tocotrienols).

Selenium, 100-200 micrograms per day.

Mixed carotenoids, 10,000-15,000 IU daily.

The antioxidants can be most conveniently taken as part of a daily multivitamin/multimineral supplement. It should contain no iron (unless you are a female and having regular menstrual periods) and no preformed vitamin A (retinol). Take these supplements with your largest meal.

Women should take supplemental calcium, preferably as calcium citrate, 500-700 milligrams a day, depending on their dietary intake of this mineral. Men should avoid supplemental calcium.

Other Measures To Consider

If you are not eating oily fish at least twice a week, take supplemental fish oil, in capsule or liquid form (two to three grams a day of a product containing both EPA and DHA). Look for molecularly distilled products certified to be free of heavy metals and other contaminants.

Talk to your doctor about going on low-dose aspirin therapy, one or two baby aspirins a day (81 or 162 milligrams).

If you are not regularly eating ginger and turmeric, consider taking these in supplemental form.

Add coenzyme Q10 (CoQ10) to your daily regimen: 60-100 milligrams of a softgel form taken with your largest meal.

If you are prone to metabolic syndrome, take alpha-lipoic acid, 100 to 400 milligrams a day.

Water

Drink pure water, or drinks that are mostly water (tea, very diluted fruit juice, sparkling water with lemon) throughout the day.

Use bottled water or get a home water purifier if your tap water tastes of chlorine or other contaminants, or if you live in an area where the water is known or suspected to be contaminated.

Table of Contents

PREFACE

This book provides you the required knowledge, data and recipes to know the basics of Paleo style and the way it will essentially remodel your life if you adopt this lifestyle. This book provides you with one in every of the foremost healthiest Paleo diet plans and following these diets can assist you to attain a lean physique and an overall healthy body and mind.

You will have additional energy throughout the day and can get much better sleep at nighttime, your skin and hair also will show a distinction in general health. This diet is additionally very straightforward to follow as you'd simply have to be compelled to eat lean meats, recent vegetables, and ocean foods. This book can show you the way to avoid ingestion modern-day foods that are extremely processed and contain colossal amounts of sugars and others have a high salt content. it'll walk you through the processes of a way to avoid sugary foods and the way to tackle the matter of sugar cravings with the assistance of paleo sugars.

Nowadays it's not regarding what quantity you're eating however in fact what you're eating and every one of that affects your health and fitness. during this present time of science and technological analysis, scientists have proved through various studies that consuming whole grains, dairy farm merchandise, and different processed foods leads to several diseases that embody polygenic disorder, heart diseases, obesity, cancer, and blood pressure.

But upon more reading you will get to know how superb Paleo diet is and the way you'll be able to incorporate it in your life to avoid all of those diseases and live a healthy life. This book can create your intake easy and assist you to melt off fat and win the lifestyle that you just desired for a long time and restore your vigor and guarantee you an extended and healthy life.

CHAPTER 1

INTRODUCTION:

The Paleo diet is the healthiest plan in the world, requiring no starvation, and no horrendous, continuous exercise. It looks to how our ancestors ate, all those thousands of years before, when things like diabetes, obesity, and heart disease did NOT rule the earth— as they do today. And, with that past diet plan, we discover a healthier way to lose weight, to prevent diseases, and to ward off serious mental issues, like depression and anxiety.

What our prehistoric ancestors ate are a few things that we won't be able to specifically verify. None people lived throughout those times and thus, it might be arduous to pinpoint specifically what they ate them. We cannot probably return in time, will we? At most, we can just build an informed however reliable guess supported no matter info we've got uncovered from the past. Supported various analysis studies, the kind of food prehistoric individuals ate were, for the most part, restricted to what was out there in their geographic locations throughout any given time. What they're are often deduced through meticulous scientific studies and advanced laboratory analysis of the prehistoric bones and dentures of Paleolithic individuals. Results from such studies served as a basis for our assumptions of what constitutes the primal diet.

We can conjointly build plausible assumptions on what constitutes the primal diet through sheer logical reasoning. By learning the kind of food we've got these days that couldn't probably have existed throughout the Paleolithic era, we must always additional or less be able to verify what style of food prehistoric individuals ever consumed through the method of elimination. By hanging out modern foodstuff that couldn't have probably existed throughout the stone-age era from our food list, we will be able to set out with a plan on what our ancestors ate.

For example,

They had no dairy farm product then as animals weren't however domesticated. it might completely be not possible and even too risky to take advantage of wild cows (if they already existed) or alternative fresh wild animals.

Agriculture wasn't existent then and thus Paleolithic individuals hardly had cereal grains. no matter grains they'll have had may are gathered from plants that grew wild within the fields that ought to be in for the most part restricted quantities.

They never salt-cured their food since they didn't have salt too at that point. There's no documentary proof existing these days that shows stone-age individuals mined salt throughout their era. the sole doable issue they might have done then was to dip their food in salt water.

Sugar wasn't however out there too at that point solely usable sweetener they would have used is wild honey that we can assume was also arduous to seek out at that time.

Lean meat from wild animals was their common menu which suggests their diet had higher protein content compared to today's diets.

Their consumption of proteins is additionally low however wealthy in fiber compared to trendy diets as their carbohydrate supply comes back from wild fruits and plants existing at that point most of that are non-starchy and thus have lower carbohydrate content.

They didn't have trans-fats like what we tend to typically get from processed foodstuff these days. What they had were omega3 fats, unsaturated fats and healthy monounsaturated fats from lean meat, fish, and food.

The Paleo diet offers an essential weight loss and healthy lifestyle plan. The diet plan works with the way your body has evolutionarily evolved to give you the food you naturally crave —the food that will help you age well, live well, and drop pounds from your waistline.

The Paleo diet may be a diet not like any other diet out there - as a result of the Paleo Diet isn't a diet!! Yeah, you heard that right. I hate the thought of a diet, and that I have a hidden suspicion that you simply do similarly. The Paleo Diet may be a fashion and once you see the light - or during this case, feel the light, you may simply surrender all those unhealthy foods permanently. I'll show you the manner and hold your hand through this journey.

Read through the book, try it, see how you feel, and evaluate your daily life and make adjustments accordingly. Every one of us is different and we all respond to foods and diets differently - Bottom line... give it a shot and see how you feel, because, at the end of the day, that's the only real science you need. Our diet and health should never be a constant thought in our minds. We eat to survive, and food is fuel for the body. Back in the days of our ancient ancestors, they didn't think about calories and fat content. The word "carbs" never came into their conversations. And yet they lived an extremely healthy and fit lifestyle and were able to have the energy necessary to hunt and gather food every day. Why is this the case? Why do you have to think so much about your daily caloric intake? It isn't about that. I want you to get 'counting calories' out of your mind right now. Once you fully grasp the idea of the Paleo lifestyle, you'll begin to see that this way of life has far more benefits than the typical American diet has to offer.

CHAPTER 2

The Paleo Diet versus the twenty-first Century Western Diet

What our prehistoric ancestors had been natural, unprocessed food that they forage or hunted inside their immediate geographic region. the trendy urban diet, on the opposite hand, is usually processed foodstuff dominated by sweetener and cereals and synthetically made ingredients. The comparison is clearly a toss-up between what's natural and what is artificial. as to which one is best, we have to shall shall shall leave this up to your personal judgment.

But what has been construed because the Paleo diet truly has 2 to 3 times more fiber than the standard average Western diet. it has twice more unsaturated fats and monounsaturated fats and 4 times more Omega three fats. A lot of important issue with this primal diet is that it's a half-hour to four-hundredth less saturated fats than the trendy urban diet. Its protein content is 2 to 3 times over the typical modern urban diet.

Since the Paleo diet contains moderate amounts of helpful fats and carbohydrates with low glycemic indexes and a load of useful phytochemicals, it's the proper diet to stop weight gain and avoid cardiac diseases. On the opposite hand, there are voluminous proofs that link the trendy urban diet to a high incidence of pandemic cardiac diseases and fatness nowadays. The monounsaturated fat content of the Paleo Diet comes principally from nuts and has been tested to guard us against cardiac diseases in a minimum of six clinical studies. The omega three fat content is additionally higher within the primal diet than in the meat from today's domesticated animals since they're grain or corn fed and not fed with polyunsaturated fatty acid rich grass. Omega three fat conjointly has cardio protecting properties. The saccharide content of the primal diet has a lower glycemic index than the carbs from modern diets since they primarily return from non-starchy fruits and vegetables. it's simply that the human body remains genetically tailored to the primal diet. whereas it's not possible to duplicate the diet specifically because it existed throughout the prehistoric era, it will serve as the rule of thumb to design effective diet interventions to guard man from the incidence of cardio diseases.

The advantages and Disadvantages of the Paleo Diet

Since the Paleo diet gained prominence, it attracted advocates additionally as detractors. Naturally, the advocates can solely sing praises and heap accolades for this new dietary plan. On the opposite hand, its detractors are going to be fast to illustrate perceived flaws in its logic. For your sake, we are enumerating here all the arguments for and against the Paleo conception coming back from each side. we will leave the ultimate decision to your higher judgment.

The advantages

Paleo diet advocates proclaim that the diet provides a bunch of great health advantages among that are:

1. The Paleo diet protects against weight gain. Since the diet prescribes solely non-starchy fruits and vegetables as its main supply of carbohydrates and not from grains and sugar that have high glycemic indexes, the hypoglycemic agent levels within the blood are down so preventing carbohydrates from being born-again and kept as fat. It truly results in important weight loss within the long run.

2. Despite having high levels of saturated fats, the Paleo diet has been shown to boost blood lipid profiles. It will increase the positive sterol (HDL) levels whereas decreasing the TG or triglycerides so, effectively shielding the heart from coronary artery disease and stroke. It conjointly has been shown to convert less dense unhealthy sterol (LPL) into high-density smart cholesterol (HDL).

3. The Paleo diet is protein free since it leaves out wheat and different cereals from wherefrom gluten are formed. It enhances digestion since the food intake is restricted to the kind of food the physical body has been acquainted with for many years.

4. The Paleo diet eliminates glucose spikes and maintains stable energy levels within the body. You typically won't get afternoon fatigues as what happens typically once you eat loads of cereals and sugar throughout the day.

5. It prevents bloating and promotes well being since there's a lot of fiber intake within the saltless diet. All of the food and beverages within the Paleo diet are organic. folks on the Paleo diet feel energetic, sleep finer, and aren't vulnerable to depression.

The disadvantages

Critics of the Paleo diet haven't wasted time to post their criticisms. Among the various objections, they need thus far printed are the following:

1. The Paleo diet is simply too tough for the easy person to follow because it entails an amazing amendment in one's fashion. it'd take herculean efforts to visualize it through to success. With such a large amount of food restrictions, it'll need changes not solely in your consumption habits

however in buying food things since you would like to pick only organic food product and meat from farm animal that has been raised and grass fed in pasture lands. it'll entail taking a better cross-check food labels to create positive they contain solely natural and organic ingredients.

2. The shift to a Paleo fashion is also dearer than usual. The fruits and vegetables ought to be organically mature and this positively can cost you higher than the regular fruits and vegetables sold-out anyplace. The meat should be from a eutherian mammal that has been grass fed or fed with corn or grains. Paleo detractors also claim that the Paleo food list includes foodstuff that isn't solely less in supply however also is costlier.

3. Critics of the Paleo diet feels that by going out grains and cereals, the diet is in result depriving the body of abundant required fiber intake and carbohydrates. They think about the Paleo as an unbalanced diet. They conjointly feel it's absurd to use modern foodstuff to structure man's original ancient diet. They believe that Paleo advocates would have a problem to remain on the diet since critics believe that because it's arduous to find strictly organic and natural food sources. They predict that Paleo advocates are about to be discouraged and are seemingly going to abandon the diet shortly once they have tried it.

- There's but, a typical ground among the advocates and also the critics of the diet. each party doesn't question the very fact that man ought to eat foods as natural and as contemporary as doable. this can be truly the terrible essence of the Paleo fashion and it seems that the higher criticisms are additionally like excuses to not adopt the diet than reasons to invalidate the effectualness of the diet.

CHAPTER 3

Correcting the Misconceptions regarding the Paleo Diet

Contrary to what the critics say, the Paleo diet is that the best and also the simplest diet to follow compared to different dietary regimens. It needs no calorie count. It simply desires a good resolve to stay to regular organic food intake and to avoid processed foodstuff and artificial ingredients. it's the healthiest too. Dieters are merely keen on creating excuses after they can't resist the urge of reversion to their recent consumption habits and succumb to the urges of their old cravings for things sweet. allow us to try and analyze the various misconceptions regarding the Paleo diet to raised appreciate its advantages.

What is the Paleo diet?

The Paleo Diet is largely a dietary idea supported on the assumption that by consuming in the like manner our stone-age ancestors did and limiting our food intake to the sort of food out there to them 2.5 million years agone, we'll become more fit, meaner, and healthier. it's over simply a bunch of well-concocted recipes. it's a full fashion that conjointly involves consuming modern food which is comparable to the food they ate and in the most state of nature attainable.
The Paleo diet isn't without any scientific basis. it's backed by historical proof, pure logic, and innumerable studies. a similar kind of transformative logic is applied to essential manner habits like sleep and exercise.

What is the underlying logic behind the Paleo diet?

The underlying logic upon that the Paleo Diet hinges based mostly on the assumption that the genetic composition of recent man has been programmed towards the diet man has been consuming since the time of our stone-age forefathers and it's not evolved a lot of since then. For over 2.5 million years, man has had a constant natural diet consisting of untamed plants and animals such a lot in order that human genetics is believed to be already programmed towards this sort of diet and therefore the agricultural and technological revolution within the last 10,000 years has hardly affected it. this can be the transformative logic on that the Paleo Diet is predicated. there's proof that our ancestors were utterly healthy as they will be and are freed from the diseases Homo sapiens suffer from nowadays. Our genes additionally as our physiology evolved from an extended process of natural decisions that created a modern human being more suited to eat the food that their genes have evolved with for various years.

How is that the Paleo diet totally different from alternative diets?

First of all, the Paleo diet isn't a reducing diet. it's property over the long run and promotes overall health and longevity. not like alternative diets, it's not targeted on achieving simply one, a specific goal like losing weight, enhancing performance in an athletic contest or just being an area of an illness management program. not like those diets, the Paleo diet promotes the health, well being, competitive performance and therefore the ideal weight of people by making hormonal balance within the body.

What is allowed and what's not allowed within the Paleo Diet?

The Paleo diet encourages the consumption of food high in useful fats significantly those from animal sources, high in animal supermolecule, and moderate intake of natural carbohydrates returning from fruits and vegetables, nuts and seeds. The useful fats ought to embody saturated fats from oil, duck fat, lard, tallow, and butter in conjunction with monounsaturated fats from avocados and vegetable oil.

Why must you get on this diet?

This is an easy, straightforward and simple to follow a diet that needs none of the cumbersome calorie numeration typical of different diets. it's the first diet humans are programmed to eat. Following this diet provides you a bevy of advantages that's unmatched by different diets. the advantages embody weight loss, muscle gain, higher digestion, stronger system, slowed aging, a lot of energy, quality sleep, less stress, better skin, and stronger teeth and bones among several different things. the most effective half is it protects you from several of the diseases of wealthiness that has infested modern humans for the last two hundred years like cardiovascular disease, diabetes, Crohn's unwellness.

What would be a typical Paleo daily diet?

You can begin your typical Paleo day with a straightforward breakfast of 2 eggs cooked in butter with almond flour muffins and a few slices of bacon. For lunch, you'll be able to have Paleo chicken fajitas or Paleo salad summer wrap rolled in a leaf of romaine lettuce. they're simple to make. For specific preparation, directions see our Paleo lunch recipes. An afternoon snack will be one or two of macadamia nuts or almonds that ever you favor otherwise you can prepare a bowl of berries mixed with some coconut milk. Dinner will be a straightforward dish of cooked asparagus and mushrooms fancy with minced contemporary rosemary springs.

Are bacon and eggs healthy?

Eggs from free travel chickens feeding on natural diets of plants and insects and bacon from grass-fed, pasture born and raised placental ought to be free from antibiotics, artificial food supplements, and growth-boosting hormones. they're natural and organic and are so healthy. Organic egg yolks and bacon contain generous quantities of useful polyunsaturated fatty acid fat and smart cholesterin. each contains healthy saturated fat that is crucial for the economical operation of just about each cell in our body. Besides, saturated fats ought to even be our main supply of calories over the carbohydrates. A modest quantity of common salt within the bacon or egg is really healthy. As for those that dislike the chemical group in bacon, there are nitrate free kinds of bacon on the market in the supermarkets. Nitrates are present compounds and may not be a priority. they will be found in a lot of higher doses in much all vegetables. "Cavemen eat this sort of diet as a result of which they are more physically active" Nothing will be clear of the reality that this story floated around by detractors of the Paleo diet. whereas it's true that the prehistoric cave dweller was a lot more physically active than the common modern human these days, he didn't eat on purpose as a result of the physical activities he engaged in. He ate to survive and whenever he may, he would conjointly realize a while to relax, take a nap, and have a decent night's sleep. The principle behind the caveman's diet is easy enough for individuals to grasp and appreciate. once you are extremely active and have interaction frequently in daily exercises, you really burn a lot of-of the sugar reserves referred to as glycogens that are stored in your muscles and liver. they have to get replaced otherwise you won't have a similar level of energy for the same activity subsequent time around. To remedy this and restore your strength and stamina you wish a lot of macromolecule intake. In different words, you'll be able to afford to possess a lot of macromolecule intake than the common person as a result of your physically active style. Corollary to the present, an individual who hardly exercises and spends most of his waking hours behind a table or on a couch look TV should eat fewer macromolecules otherwise any excess carbohydrate intake are going to be regenerate and keep as fat leading to weight gain and ultimately fatness that threatens to shorten your existence on earth.

Why is sugar prohibited within the Paleo Diet once it's really natural?

Sure enough, sugar is usually a present substance. we discover it in virtually everything nature produces. However, once it's refined into focused granules or powder and used intrinsically like we tend to do these days it becomes poison to the physical structure. it's now not in its natural diluted type. Continuous consumption of sugar will cause spikes in blood glucose levels which can induce strokes or result in other health issues like polygenic disorder. Fruits are the foremost ideal sources of sugar and carbohydrates as a result of the absorption of sugar from the fruits we tend to eat is tempered and over-involved by its high fiber content. Besides, the vitamins, phytonutrients, and antioxidants within the fruit stop injury to the cells once the sugar is oxidized at the cellular level. They additionally repair no matter damage could have already been done to the cells as a result of the reaction of sugar. we've full-grown accustomed to obtaining our sugar fix by adding teaspoon jam-packed with sugar to the food we tend to eat and also the beverages we drink while not realizing we are inflicting heavy injury to our own bodies. it's time we tend to get our sugar fix from a lot of natural sources like fruits. it's safer and healthier that means.

Cavemen died young, therefore why do we tend to adopt their diet?

Again, this can be another one in each of the numerous myths being floated around by detractors to discredit the Paleo diet. the reality is there's proof that shows that our Paleolithic ancestors lived longer than what the majority thought. several of them who died young, died within the hands of different predators or by being gored by their own prey whereas on a pursuit. Others died of starvation or accidents, however, hardly any of them died of natural cause or health problems. the sole reason why modern humans live longer these days is as a result of he has access to advanced medical aid and technology and not as a result of his diet. Infectious diseases will currently be for the most part contained and neutralized. while not trendy medical facilities individuals these days would die early. And, on the contrary, there's mounting proof linking the fashionable urban diet to such life-threatening health conditions like cardiovascular disease, cancer, excretory organ and liver issues, diabetes, and different diseases of affluence.

How am I able to keep Paleo notwithstanding I dine out often?

If you're on the Paleo diet, you must not have any worries if you've got to travel and get on the road for some time. Neither must you worry if you suddenly commit to treating yourself or your family or friends to dinner out of a whim. you'll be able to keep Paleo wherever ever you go. the sole hurdle would be you - however resolute you're in sticking to the Paleo style no matter you are doing, wherever ever you go, and whichever state of affairs you'll end up in. within the 1st place, there are Paleo friendly restaurants scattered everywhere the country and their variety are on the increase. You shouldn't have a problem finding one to eat in. it's not such a lot just like the previous days wherever you'd seldom realize restaurants that serve protein free and strictly organic dishes. Today, protein free and organic is the 'in' factor among restaurants from the high finish elegant restaurants to the regular sustenance chains and mall food retailers. These Paleo-friendly restaurants are germination like mushrooms everywhere in the country and in several major cities all over the globe. There are even Paleo food trucks roaming around some cities serving strictly Paleo dishes on the enter street corners and parking tons. Before you continue a visitor before you eat with friends and family, build it a habit to see out that Paleo-friendly restaurants are settled in the area wherever you propose to travel. List down these restaurants before you permit the house for the trip or the planned dinner with friends or family. Don't live the house while not this list. you'll be able to do an internet search for Paleo-friendly buildings or check our restaurant list during this eBook. There could also be times you'll end up during a state of affairs wherever you get invited by friends to eat in a non-Paleo friendly building. Don't be back to raise the waiter if they need protein free dishes. At a similar time feint an excuse why you wish your meal to be protein free like having a heavy hypersensitivity reaction to grains and meals with traces of grain in them will be fatal to you. you'll be able to make sure they'll take this seriously as a result of if there's something building owners worry most it's having a client develop a health condition as a result of their food. Oh, and don't forget to inform them to not use oil in the preparation of your meal. Feint a similar 'allergy' excuse. follow your Paleo diet even once eating out with friends in restaurants or once you get invited for dinner in their homes. Don't desire the 'odd man out' once you refuse some food. However, once you refuse a number of the foods they serve you wish to elucidate why so that they won't feel slighted. simply make a case for that what you refused could do some injury to your health. you'll be able to take this chance to debate with them the Paleo diet and also the advantage of eating healthy. who knows? you'll nonetheless win them over to the Paleo style. And notwithstanding they don't convert to Paleo you'll be able to a minimum of making sure that subsequent time they invite you over they'll prepare one thing that's Paleo for you.

Should I be going back to a traditional diet when I reach my targeted weight?

Many people who press on a diet desires to slenderize most in order that they assume that each one forms of special diet Paleo included is merely for losing weight. To them, something with the word 'diet' has become synonymous with weight loss. However, the Paleo diet is quite simply a weight loss formula. it's not one thing you ought to discard when achieving your ideal weight. it's instead a formula for a healthy manner that you would have to embrace for the remainder of your life if you would like a disease-free, healthier body and an extended lifespan. Besides, it makes no sense to travel back to a diet that within the initial place is that the main reason for your being overweight. Of course, you absolve to do as you want together with going back to your recent consumption habits and exposing yourself all over again to heart diseases, diabetes, and different modern-day afflictions that hounds man these days. It's your choice however make it sensible. If you have got reached your ideal weight on the Paleo diet it suggests that it's effective and there's a lot of reason currently to remain on with it. however please note that weight loss is simply a part of the helpful effects of this diet. it'll heal the harm done by a trendy urban diet has done to your gut and still balance the hormones in your system. this may take it slow to realize which suggests you continue to keep doing Paleo even long after reaching your ideal weight. Anyway, if you keep Paleo for a few time you'll get accustomed to it and notice it not solely delicious however additionally fulfilling.

Shouldn't we tend to eat meat the manner the cavemen did?

The ideal Paleo diet ought to embrace each raw and prepared meat. there's but a sub-category of Paleo adherents who believe that consumption solely raw Paleo meat is that the ideal diet. The decision it Raw Paleo. Their variety remains little, however, it's growing. On the opposite hand, the bulk of Paleo advocates value more highly to have their meat prepared. it might be incorrect to mention that cavemen invariably ate their meat raw. maybe they did before they found the way to begin starting fire. however once man learned the way to begin starting a fire he additionally learned to cook the food he ate. And there's overwhelming proof that dates for several years to prove he did. preparation makes meat a lot of eatables and absorbed by our systems. whereas it's true that preparation destroys abundant of the meat's nutrients, it properly compensates for this by making prepared meat simply eatable and extremely absorbable. no matter nutrients are left within the prepared meat, they simply reach each a part of the body together with the brain, nourishing and dashing up their growth and development within the whole process. it's no surprise then why man's brain developed quicker than those of the remainder of the kingdom. Our brain is greater than those of the opposite animal species and this can be as a result of the learned to cook the food he ate that made the food easier to digest and also the nutrients promptly out there to be used by each cell within the physical body. It wouldn't be, however, to assume that our Paleo ancestors prepared their food as extensively as we tend to do these days. At the onset, they have to have tried experimenting with it and their diet must have been a mixture of prepared and meat. Certainly, there's space for meat within the modern Paleo diet. actually, the optimum Paleo diet ought to be a mixture of raw and done. And if you don't have the abdomen for meat, you'll be able to at least cook it rare or medium-rare. Or, you'll be able to eat raw fish and home-cured dishes for a change in food.

How much fat, proteins and carbs do I eat?

Unless you're an endurance athlete exercising in preparation for an athletic event, there's no enumeration of calories or activity of fat, protein, or sugar intake for your Paleo diet. And albeit you're an athlete there's no atomic number or quantitative relation of food intake that everybody should follow to achieve optimum results the Paleo diet. what proportion fat, protein, and carbohydrates an individual desire depends on his individual needs and private circumstance. just in case you haven't noticed, the dietary recommendations of every one among those promoting the diet differs slightly from each other. There are hardly any 2 recommendations that are precisely alike once it involves suggested dietary intake. this can be as a result of completely different people who have different physical build, health condition, personal preferences, and fitness objects. Some merely prefer to slenderize. Others are a lot of into rigid physical learning in readiness for future athletic competitions. There also are people who are into the Paleo diet as a part of a health maintenance program to cure reaction diseases. Naturally, the nutrient demand depends on individual needs which is able to not be similar to those of the opposite people with completely different requirements or nutritionary needs. Certainly, the Paleo diet isn't any remedy or a cure resolution for people who would like to pursue a healthy manner or no matter their objectives perhaps. Paleo isn't sort of a 'one size fits all' form of a diet. And, the best approach to following the diet is to simply eat no matter is natural and organic together with tons of helpful animal fats. The safest combination ought to be high fat, low carbohydrates, and moderate supermolecule. But again, how high is 'high' and the way low is 'low' can depend upon individual desires and needs. There are extremely no rules written on a stone for individuals to follow. you will adopt a selected Paleo diet recommendation however you may have to be compelled to check that changes to suit your personal preference or style. however so long as what you eat is natural and organic and belongs to the Paleo food list, it'll still be Paleo. The Paleo diet for endurance contestants may be a completely different story particularly if the athlete is on to a rigorous coaching regime. in step with good shape coaches a contestant who ought to consume two hundred to three hundred calories from straightforward to digest sugar sources an hour before his scheduled exercise with another 200 to 300 calories each hour thenceforth for the length of his work out. He additionally needs to take another two hundred to three hundred calories within a half-hour when the exercise to assist the body to recover from the strenuous workout.

Are supplements allowed?

Doctors would unremarkably advocate supplements to persons with specific health conditions in line with severe victuals deficiencies otherwise they'd instead recommend a diet made within the deficient vitamins or minerals. The Paleo diet is already dense in vitamins and minerals that the body desires. Unless the deficiency is serious enough to want 'shock treatment supplements are whole extra. Besides, most supplements are synthetically created. Or, they'll return from organic extracts however they still contain artificial ingredients. they will do a lot of damage than good to your body within the long run. If you're on the Paleo diet there's no more need for supplements. it'll simply be a waste of your cash since the diet has all the nutrients you would like. All you would like to try and do is stick with the diet and let it heal your body naturally – while not supplements. provides it a decent time to figure your body and heal it from years of injury caused by the food you've been consuming. In time your gut can finally have the best secretion balance it has to operate expeditiously. If you're from a northern county or work inside most of the time likelihood is that you are vitamin d deficient. go out under the sun more typically and for extended periods. You'll get all the vitamin d you require from daylight. what's good is that it's free.

Is there a settling time period to the Paleo diet?

Weaning over to the Paleo diet from your recent diet might} would like may need an adjustment period of nearly three to four weeks. it's no joke to form a fast shift to a less carb diet once your body is so accustomed to being bombarded with high carb doses every day for several years. you will encounter some lightheadedness or feel lightsome most of the time. you will even be jittery and irritable. These are traditional bodily reactions if you begin taking under fifty grams of carbohydrates that is all that the Paleo diet can provide you with every single day. however, don't worry as a result of these withdrawal symptoms can presently glide by. And as you get accustomed to the diet more and more on a daily basis, you may begin to feel extremely energized. The Paleo diet features a detoxing result on your body. It starts to urge obviate the toxins that have accumulated in your muscles cells of these years. These toxins are discharged to the bloodstream and ultimately excreted out of your body by your system. you may be experiencing detoxing symptoms like lightheadedness or irritability throughout this stage however this can be solely temporary. you may solely feel such symptoms whereas the diet remains cleansing your body and subsequently you will feel energetic and active.

How much concerned should I be regarding withdrawal symptoms?

You may undergo alkaloid withdrawal headaches or the alleged 'low carb flu' manifested in ways that like feeling weak, feeling tired, having headaches, or alternatively equally light-weight symptoms. you don't need need to not worry because they're going to disappear in a matter of a few days. simply stay resolute and follow the diet. everybody who switched over to the Paleo diet perpetually become to be grateful as a result of the discomfort they went through for a brief amount of time was nothing compared to the immeasurable advantages they gained from it.

How long can it take before I begin feeling accustomed on a Paleo diet?

After fourteen to thirty days on the diet, the typical person ought to begin feeling the total useful effects of going Paleo. Of course, this might vary from person to person reckoning on how they strictly follow the diet. If you go strict Paleo right from day one you will undergo more intense however shorter detoxing syndromes. But, you'll feel far better from the fourteenth day and onwards.

Aren't fish and food dangerous owing to high levels of mercury in them?

Fish or any food for that matter that has high levels of mercury is unsafe to your health. this can be very true for industrially created farmed fish or those who are raised in fish pens or cages. However, the reality is fish caught wild from the ocean has less mercury content than the vegetables we tend to purchase from the market. Fish ought to be an integral part of the Paleo Diet as a result of it's the most effective supply of high levels of Omega three. that's why in the coming time you purchase fish you must check the labels to know for certain it's not farmed fish however fish caught from the ocean. the higher possibility is to shop for fish from the fisherman's wharf if you reside close to one.

Is the Paleo diet a mere fashionable diet?

The Paleo diet is over-programmed food intake. it's a complete style that revolves around uptake solely natural and organic foodstuff. It can't be a fashion since this type of diet has been existing for innumerable years. it's property for a lifespan and not one thing individuals will simply lose interest as time goes by.

Isn't this similar to Atkins?

Many people erroneously suppose, therefore. On the onset, they sometimes do look similar however if you cross-check them closely you'll discover that there are vital variations between the 2 that sets them apart. For one factor, the Paleo diet permits you to eat as several contemporary fruits as you wish – no restrictions whereas Atkins solely allows controlled servings and not all fresh fruits are allowed. however, the foremost vital distinction between the 2 is that the proven fact that the Atkins diet permits the consumption of heaps of processed meats and saturated fats. The Paleo diet, on the opposite hand, bans all processed meats and puts stress on animal macromolecule and useful fats from grass-fed, free from farm animals solely.

Can the Paleo Diet assist you to lose weight?

The simple answer is affirmative. Weight loss is, however, a positive residual result of the Paleo diet. Its real price is keeping you healthy, fit, and feeling such a lot better for the long-term. don't expect it to be a fast fix for weight gain. you'll slim down o.k. however, it won't be very dramatic. Rather, it'll be a gradual method that creates it extremely manageable and actually long term and a lot of permanent. With the Paleo diet, the body is instructed to use fat for energy and limit its dependence on carbohydrates for energy. within the method, there'll hardly be any excess fat to behold on and no matter fat is there will be regenerate into energy to power cell functions. you furthermore may get to avoid high supermolecule intake which may cause spikes in glucose levels. rock bottom line is that the majority of individuals who adopted the Paleo diet achieved vital weight loss once being within the diet for a considerable time. the great news is it forever corrects the body's dependence on carbohydrates and you'd be able to maintain your ideal weight with hardly any effort.

What am I able to get from following the Paleo Diet?

Weight loss is one among a lot of vital edges you'll gain from following the diet. There are heaps of other different edges it provides like progressing to sleep far better at night, improved skin complexion, improved sex drive (if you would like to think about it significant), improved digestion, clearer mind, and inflated energy. The Paleo diet heals your body back to its original condition very like overhauling an automotive and repairing broken components. It will cure such diseases as Crohn's disease and alternative response diseases.

Won't you get bored consuming virtually identical foods each day?

Theoretically, the solution would be affirmative you will get bored. The Paleo diet doesn't have an in-depth line of luxurious recipes as what you have got been accustomed for years and should taste otherwise with sugar and salt deliberately disregarded. however, if you think about the actual fact that our body appearance for selection solely as a result of it's not obtaining the best nutrition from the food you eat then you'll better appreciate and perceive why Paleo converts are sticking out to the diet permanently. Your decisions of food on the Paleo diet are also restricted however they offer you the best nutrition that ultimately curves your cravings for selection. Besides, it's not true that the Paleo lacks selection. The Paleo recipes enclosed during this book are simply some of the numerous Paleo dishes you'll notice around. and that they are by no means that less luxurious. individuals tend to consider the Paleo diet as another one among those bland and tasteless slimming diets. Nothing will be clear of the reality and therefore the thousands of recipes you'll discover online is proof of this. you'll have a range of healthy foods while not venturing out of the Paleo tips. whereas several prefer to follow an easy diet, you'll elect to possess a selection in your Paleo meals and an easy online search can assist you to do this with ease.

Why do I need to avoid adding salt to my food?

Intake of salt additionally as grains, legumes, and cheese creates an extremely acidic setting in our bodies and puts tremendous stress on our kidneys. As a reaction response, the body is forced to trigger the calcium reserves in our bones to neutralize the acidity and restore balance all over again. the total result of this, however, ends up in chronic diseases like pathology.

Grains have fibers, minerals, and vitamins, therefore, why ought to I take it out from my diet?

The little identified truth regarding whole grains is that they contain an indigestible substance referred to as phytate that stores energy and therefore the part phosphorous within the grain. Phytate is that the salt sort of phytic acid that binds the metallic element, iron, zinc, and calcium in our intestines and effectively leading them out of our bodies preventing them from being absorbed by our system. Mammals {including|as we tend toll as|together with} humans cannot digest phytate, as a result, we don't have the catalyst phytase. without that, it can't be digestible or absorbed leaving it to wreck mayhem by obstructing the much-needed nutrients we mentioned on top of from being absorbed by the body. This in result makes grains anti-nutrients. we tend to do need fiber in our diet fruits and vegetables will give the fibers we'd like. Fruits and vegetables are healthier sources of fibers than grain that do a lot of injury than benefit to our bodies. in contrast to the fibers found in grains, the fiber in fruits and vegetables is very soluble and is well assimilated into our system while not doing injury to the walls of the intestines that grain fibers notoriously do. On top of all that, fruits and vegetables contain a lot of B vitamins and folacin than grain. It won't add up to continue eating grain that has fewer nutrients and does a lot of injury to our system once we will get more nutrients from healthy sources like fruits and vegetables without having to risk damaging to our intestines.

Can a vegetarian get on Paleo Diet at the same time?

The simple answer to this question is no. they need to settle on between the 2 as a result of the basic distinction that prevents them from a combination like water and oil. as an example, most vegetarians rely heavily on the utilization of grains and legumes like beans, peas, as their main supply of carbohydrates for his or her daily calorie necessities. As you well grasp by now grains and legumes don't seem to be allowed within the Paleo diet. they're anti-nutrients and cause chronic inflammation of the intestines a condition known as leaky gut that may be a precursor to several problems such as heart diseases also as cancer. Besides that, a strict feeder diet deprives the body of the much-needed nutrients, vitamins, and minerals that are unremarkably found packed in animal food sources. The feeder diet specifically ends up in deficiencies in vitamins D, B6, and B12 and essential minerals like iron, zinc, and iodine and useful nutrients like omega three fatty acids and taurine.

Is the paleo diet reaching to punch a hole in my pocket?

It is an incontrovertible fact that processed foods created in giant quantities are cheaper than organically grown fresh foods. There is not a single doubt that the Paleo diet is going to be pricier than processed foods. However, if you're thinking that of the long run then let me tell you that it is going to free you from the travails of the fashionable urban diet and prevent from future medical expenses you're seeming to incur once you get afflicted with the numerous diseases as a result of prolonged consumption of processed food. In the end, you're probably going to be paying a lot on medical bills than the cash you saved by shopping for cheaper processed foods.

Is it sensible to bring a Paleo pack lunch to work?

A packed lunch consisting of a vegetable dish flat-topped with grilled pigeon breast is simple to organize. Add an apple or a bag of nuts and pack some vegetables and you have got an ideal lunch to travel with. And if you don't have the time to organize a meal yourself you'll be able to attempt the prepacked Paleo meals that are currently obtainable from many online sources and in several selections. simply heat up it during a microwave at your office and you have got a hot, healthy lunch.

Do I actually have to travel to a specialty food store to shop for my Paleo foodstuff?

Natural organic foods aren't solely obtainable in specialty outlets like monger Joe's. they will be found even in your neighborhood grocery store. you simply got to scan the labels rigorously. If you wish to make certain what you're obtaining is natural and organic then create it a habit to go to the farmer's market close to you. You'll get them contemporary there. For organic meat and poultry, the most effective manner is to induce them directly from certified producers. you'll be able to try this by a change of integrity any Community Supported Agriculture organization. I'm positive there's one close to you. Not solely are you able to make certain that you just can you get your meat and poultry from organically raised and grass-fed placental, however, you'd even be able to get them contemporary and at remarkably cheaper costs.

Is it an occasional carb, fad diet?

Critics say the Paleo Diet is simply another reducing diet that's low in carbohydrates and so unbalanced. Nothing may be clear of the reality that this unwarranted allegation. The Paleo diet isn't low in carbohydrates. Rather, its saccharide content has low glycemic indices since they are available from non-starchy fruits and vegetables. there's an enormous deal of distinction between having low macromolecule content and having carbohydrates that have low glycemic indexes. The Paleo diet encourages you to consume loads of fiber made fruits and vegetables that are its main sources of carbohydrates for energy. the trendy urban diet on the opposite hand depends on loads on sugar and cereals for energy that sadly causes spikes in glucose levels. It can't be reducing diet either as a result of man has been consuming this sort of diet even long before the appearance of agriculture. it's really man's survival diet since it's been able to exist on this diet disease-free for many years.

Is it tough to follow?

The most important issue regarding Paleo is that the incontrovertible fact that it entails no guesswork and needs no calorie count and constant observation. it's a no-fuss dietary arrange that doesn't need you to perpetually make mathematical calculations or dine in the zone to make certain you're not overstepping through programmed dietary food intake.

CHAPTER 3

Blending your twenty-first CENTURY way to the Paleo Diet

One of the foremost tough things in incorporating changes to your 21 st Century way is in adapting the aforementioned changes to interchange established habits that don't change well to the new lifestyle. you wish to acknowledge which of them are often harmful to your efforts to attain healthiness and well being, therefore, you'll be able to do one thing to result in the changes. Here are a number of them:

If you're a tea or coffee lover and taking your morning coffee has become a daily ritual, you'll be able to plow ahead with it however you want to prune on sugar and cream. higher still take it strictly black low – no cream and sugar the least bit.

If your work keeps you busy all the time, you must survey the world around your office and establish the food shops that serve Paleo sort of foodstuff. never leave this to likelihood because if you do your set up can fail since you're probably to patronize non-Paleo food shops once hunger pangs get the higher of you before you'll be able to realize a building that's Paleo friendly.

If you slow down once to your cravings for the standard} food then you're probably to travel back to your old consumption habits and destroy your Paleo set up altogether.

If you're a cake and pastry enthusiast, you have got to give up your appetence. sweetener and farm merchandise don't have any place within the Paleo diet. you wish to work arduous to eliminate sweetener and flour from your way.

Remember that there's no area for compromise once you embrace the Paleo diet. Neither ought to there be the area for flexibility because it will destroy the diet utterly since you'll begin losing management over your consumption habits. If you're a fanatical social creature, you want to additionally prune on your nightlife or abandon it altogether. a really active social life opens you to a lot of temptations which can probably force you to interrupt your Paleo diet. Don't eat food that uses oil, corn oil, soy oil or different oils made of grains and seeds. Restaurant food sometimes makes use of those oils and thus ought to even be avoided. Butter, lard and animal oil, unrefined copra oil, and vegetable oil ought to be used instead. don't be misled by claims that saturated fats are dangerous for your health. they're smart for your heart and your overall health. We shall be discussing this during a separate section. Keep a tab on what you eat a day. begin your food diary and record not solely the food you eat but additionally, however you felt once every food intake. the info can assist you still adapt to the Paleo way a lot of simply. Our prehistoric ancestors never had an equivalent flood of food temptations you'll be featured with after you try and amendment over to the Paleo way. they'd no alternative attributable to their very existence relied on it.

Besides, it had been the sole factor they'd so it wasn't onerous for them. The twenty-first Century man, on the opposite hand, includes a ton of tempting food selections to pick from every single day. He must, therefore, be ready to create concessions and may be willing to allow up to a number of his favorite food things if he's actually serious in adopting the healthy Paleo way.

Adapting to the Paleo mode

Eat just like a cave dweller

Adapting the Paleo mode to your own involves feeding the way the cavemen of prehistoric times did. No, it's not regarding moving within a cave and feeding there. it's not regarding scavenging or trying to find your own food since you'll use modern food as a substitute. It is regarding consuming modern food that may not cause endocrine spikes. A spike in endocrine within the blood really tricks our body to store energy as fat leading to weight gain. It is quite unfortunate that the fashionable man's diet is loaded with sugar and refined cereals. many of us these days are actually therefore accustomed to taking cereals for breakfast, packed sandwiches for lunch, and completely different food preparations for dinner. They even usually supplement this with snacks in between meals consisting of fries, chips, and soda. They couldn't care less about whether or not or not the continued consumption of processed food made in sweetener and cereals can create them gain weight quickly, and over time it's going to even cause polygenic disease or within the worst case situation to cancer. Another issue that took to modern day man's current difficulty is his mistaken belief on what represents a healthy diet. folks are brainwashed to believe that consuming low-fat foods high in carbohydrates can facilitate keep the heart healthy furthermore as stop weight gain. This thought is really the offender. it's not intaking less fat and lowering carb intake which can forestall endocrine spikes. You'll solely be starving the body of abundant required nutrients that approach. The primal diet corrects this thought with a diet that contains a lot of healthy fats and non-starchy fruits and vegetables instead. it's not regarding limiting fat intake. it's regarding avoiding the utilization of trans fat and harmful omega-6 fatty acid fats from soy oil or vegetable oil that modern humans are utilizing extensively in preparing their food every single day.

Going Primal needs Resolve

One should have the correct mental attitude before adopting the Paleo mode. it's essential that one should be resolute to avoid reverting into your previous rotten ways. Primal living is over a diet or a physical exercise program – it's a complete mode amendment.
You need to understand the importance of feeding and acquiring ways in which our body is optimally designed. And it needs one to be unwavering once he starts going primal. it'll mean abandoning several things you've fully grown comfy with. it'd be like turning yourself far away from what used to be your ease zone and recharging yourself with a brand new Paleo mode. you furthermore may be a lot of physically active. One of the sick effects of progress is it had made man lazy and quite less physically active such a lot in contrast to our prehistoric ancestors who are perpetually on the move trying to find food or looking for ways in which to shield themselves from the weather. Modern human beings spend the foremost a part of his waking time sitting in a workplace or look tv reception. Every day he'd ride his automobile to figure. Weekends are holy to him because it is that the solely time during a week he sometimes comes to life late and not worry regarding being late for work. Modern human being has chosen to adopt a way of life that really slowly erodes his muscular health and ends up in cardiovascular degeneration. He must break

from the labor of his day to day routine by going out underneath the sun more than he does and doing physical exercises.

CHAPTER 4

What you have to give Up To Be Paleo

So far, you recognize that you simply have to be compelled to surrender sweetener and cereals furthermore as legumes to be Paleo. however, there is more stuff you have to be compelled to surrender once you embrace the Paleo mode. Sacrifices can have to be compelled to be made together with venturing out of what accustomed be your comfort zone and preceding several things you love and are familiar with having. Among the items you have got to give up are the following:

1. Avoid junk food chains

Fast food and most different processed food material are high in trans fat and omega-6 fatty acid fats that cause inflammation. If hamburger and fries became a part of your routine, it's time to shed the habit. Stop creating holidays as food events Christmas, Thanksgiving, Easter, Birthdays, Anniversaries, etc. have forever been a food event. we've been at home with celebrating such events by making ready luxurious meals. it'll be tough to interrupt tradition however this must be left behind for you to be Paleo. inside a food fest, you should recommend a trek to the park or something else.

2. Walk more, Ride less

Your feet are created for walking. attempt to walk as usually as you're able to and whenever time permits. Leave your automotive behind whenever you'll and walk instead. Don't take the elevators and use the steps. it's smart for your heart. no matter ways in which you'll incorporate walking or any physical exercises to your leisurely fashionable mode aiming to be|are} a welcome amendment and is unquestionably going to boost your health.

3. Resist the urge

It is extremely tough to eat otherwise from the remainder of your friends. you will feel alienated or odd and therefore the temptation to allow in and eat non-Paleo food with them is just compelling. However, there aren't any if's and but's with the Paleo mode and would have to resist all the urges and instances of yet again splurging on an unhealthy diet. Think of your own health within the next 10 years. Be robust in your resolve and you will even gain your friends' respect for your new mode.

4. Prepare yourself for the future

Never assume that Paleo could be a miracle answer to uncontrollable weight gain. If you expect to lose pounds night long you will find yourself unsuccessful. it's a way of life that you wish to embrace for the remainder of your life. The results might not be dramatic however they're going to certainly come. {they may|they'll|they can} not be immediate however positive results will come back and therefore the changes are permanent.

5. Don't take medicine to cure your symptoms

Throw all the medications within the house out of the window. If your doctor forever prescribes medicine for any symptom, it's best to contemplate trying to find another one. keep in mind that what ails man is usually connected to the type of food he takes and this is often one thing your doctor should take into account. If you are taking up the Paleo challenge, you may really facilitate yourself get eliminate these symptoms. you only got to be firm and resolute in adopting this new model.

6. Stop being a creature of habit

If you accustomed to bring out the children to eat out in some fancy restaurant chain each weekend or cook for them pancakes once they come back from college, it's time to interrupt the routine and prepare a lot of natural, healthier meals now around.

7. provide no excuses

One of the common excuses individuals use to justify feeding food is a hectic operating schedule. Drop the reasons. it's time to create firm changes on your food decisions if you want to pursue your health and fitness goals seriously.

8. head to the Farmers Market Instead

You may not be able to avoid getting to the grocery store for your house desires however take care to avoid the center section wherever most of the junk foods are. better still, you must visit the farmers' market close to you more than usual than the grocery store. They'll have many contemporary fruits and vegetables for you there.

9. Get a lot of Shine from the Sun

Don't avoid standing in the sun. it's healthy for you. Go outdoors as usually as you're able to. there's no more nutrient source for vitamin D than from sunshine.

10. reduce your dependence on fashionable gadgets

Instead of losing sleep browsing information superhighway or taking part in online games along with your iPad in bed, tuck it away and have a decent night's rest. rather than cardiopulmonary exercise or running around on specially designed shoes which will absorb shock, run barefoot. Weird because it could appear however it's extremely healthy for your body.

CHAPTER 5

What are the fundamentals of Paleo diet?

The Paleo Diet is essentially a dietary construct engineered on the idea that by intake in the like manner our stone-age ancestors did and limiting our food intake to the kind of food on the market to them then, we are going to become healthy, leaner, and healthier. It's simply a bunch of well-concocted recipes. it's a full lifestyle that conjointly involves consuming the simple food in the most natural state. The Paleolithic era is what's unremarkably said because of the stone-age era. It marked that amount within the prehistoric human history wherever man started learning the way to craft varied tools out of stone. The word 'Paleolithic' comes from 2 Greek words that mean "Old age of the stone" or Stone Age for brief. it had been additionally the time once men discovered the way to build hearth and commenced change of state the food they Ate. it had been an associate era that began regarding a pair of 6 million years past and all over simply 10,000 years past amount once agriculture and animal farming became notable to man.

It is, for the most part, believed that individuals throughout the stone-age era were primarily hunter-gatherers who survived by adornment along in tiny teams to hunt wild animals and gather edible wild plants for subsistence. These prehistoric men survived on minimally processed natural food for countless years and also the physical body was thought to own custom-made to that absolutely. The human ordering is believed to own evolved already programmed to urge its nutrients from natural sources when overwhelming identical minimally processed food for countless years. The advent of agriculture and agriculture simply 10,000 years past has brought profound changes to the manner individuals ate and also the kind of food that they had. As man's information grew, they additionally learned alternative ways to supply and method food a lot of expeditiously. Food began to be processed in ever increasing scale quickly commutation natural food sources with that man has been wont to for countless years. the commercial revolution that ensued within the same era.

In order to completely perceive how this lifestyle amendment goes to assist you within the long-term, it's essential that you just perceive the fundamental core elements of the foods you eat. Now, I promise that I'll create this as fascinating as possible, however, it's vital that you simply perceive these elements because this is often what's progressing to structure the core of your diet. We're progressing to set out with one amongst my favorite groups: proteins.

Proteins

Proteins are one of the core sources of life, they are responsible for the growth of our nails, hairs, and muscles. They also act with a lot of other enzymes and hormones in our body and have been a great source of energy for humans since the start of human life on Earth. They are present meat, eggs, fish and some vegetables and the humans have been utilizing them from the start to support their growth. They are also responsible for making our muscles grow and giving us the strength to do work. There are two kinds of proteins namely top shelf proteins and bottom shelf proteins and both of these have their benefits for the human body. In the Paleo lifestyle Proteins play a vital role and hence they cannot be neglected. They will form the basis of your new paleo lifestyle.

Carbohydrates

If you're an Olympic contestant, carbohydrates are a vital part of your diet. And if you're an athlete or muscle-builder, carbohydrates also can be a vital bit of your diet. the matter, however, is that society has outlined carbohydrates in such a way that provides them a foul name when in reality they're a vital a part of our diet - when utilized in the proper manner. That last bit is essential because carbohydrates will be used into 2 separate teams, quite like proteins. while not obtaining too technical on you, we've got monosaccharides and disaccharides. "Mono" merely means that one sugar and "di" simply means 2 sugars. this is often why we are progressing to focus on the carbohydrates that'll truly facilitate your body to improve energy levels and help your digestion at a similar time. We'll get into the various sorts of carbs in a bit.

Insulin

One of the most important indicators of fat storage needs to do with the internal secretion we tend to call insulin. you'll have heard of the term 'insulin' thrown around before on TV or seen it on the net - and there's a decent reason for it. insulin is essential in controlling your glucose levels, your body fat, and conjointly deals with aging factors. to measure an extended and spirited life, we want to give in our best to keep our insulin levels on the low aspect by controlling the foods we tend to put in our body - specifically, carbohydrates that tend to spike insulin and cause your body to store fat. to grasp insulin, we've got to additionally inspect insulin's role in controlling our glucose levels. Insulin's primary role is to inform the nutrients you set into your body where to be kept. If you're perpetually golf stroke high saccharide meals and sugar-coated foods into your system, your insulin levels spike and your body tells itself to store that energy as fat. this is often why the Paleo style avoids such foods and permits your body to the method itself and regulates insulin levels with efficiency.

GRAINS!

When you make the jump and choose to undertake Paleo or dive in full time, it's vital that you just perceive the one essential ingredient you would like to eliminate from your diet - Grains. Grains embody everything from Barley wheat, corn, oats, rice and so on. however as comfy as you're feeding these items, it's vital to understand that grains are way less nutrient than traditional vegetables, fruits, nuts, and proteins. Grains have a name for stimulating improper liver, thyroid, and duct gland responses in many folks which might, in turn, result in reduced immunity, fungal infections, skin issues, anxiety, depression, and weight gain. one amongst the issues with grains is that they inhibit the body from properly digesting them. This goes back to the means that they were evolved as a plant species with no defense reaction. Our bodies simply aren't adapted to digest these sorts of grains - period.

When you compare grains calorie for-calorie to different natural foods such as lean meats, seafood, and veggies, you perceive that they're an away weaker form of calorie and not appropriate for sustained energy. And this suggests that you just can't eat stuff like quinoa. I do know plenty of individuals out there have found quinoa to be an alternate to whole-grains, however, those don't fly, as well. because they're within the same family as grains, they still have identical forms of side effects on the digestive system as a grain. the most important issue you've got to stress concerning is that the mayhem they make on your digestive system. they have an inclination to cause what's referred to as malabsorption that, in turn, affects your health and well-being. Let's re-examine a couple of-of the problems associated with making an attempt to soak up grains in your diet:

1. For starters, grains have the tendency to break the liner of the gut. once the gut is broken, your ability to soak up nutrients is greatly diminished. we want the healthy lining of our abdomen to

soak up all the nutrients we need for our bodies. This includes all proteins, fats, carbs, vitamins, and minerals.

2. there's additionally the danger for the gall bladder to be broken. this may inhibit the production of digestive juice, which suggests we are going to not be ready to absorb essential nutrients like vitamins A, D, and K. If you can't absorb these vitamins, then you're going to have a problem absorbing essential nutrients that you just do would like.

3. Once your gut lining goes, it opens the door for pathology deficiencies and cancer. Not Good. The exocrine gland is particularly full of inflammation caused by grains passing through. this could cause carcinoma or inflammation of the exocrine gland.

4. Bottom line is... grains

aren't meant for the body and may cause digestive system issues, which can, in turn, result in additional serious issues like degenerative disorder, atrophic arthritis, lupus, vitiligo, narcolepsy, autism, and a range of different diseases. Now, I do know you'll be saying, "But, I don't have any of those diseases!" I do know, however you've got to grasp that over time, these are the problems that arise after we don't look out of our bodies and expeditiously fuel them with the proper nutrients and whole foods.

Gluten

Gluten comes from the Latin word for "glue" that is that the 1st clue that this ingredient shouldn't be placed into the bod. protein could be a form of supermolecule that's found in wheat, rye oats, and barley, and it's the ingredient that helps the dough rise and provides the food its bouncy consistency. we aren't reaching to dive deep into what protein is, however, I would like you to understand it isn't smart for any folks, and it's vital to eliminate it from your diet. I'm not reaching to beat around the bush... whether or not you would like to listen to it or not, grains aren't that healthy for you. I do know I same it! of these foods style smart. The bread, pasta, cookies, you name it – they're all extraordinarily delicious. however, you've got to see past your style buds for one second so as to induce to the important truth of the matter and to grasp what foods can truly help you live and not kill you. Let's dive into the anatomy of grain to actually comprehend it. All grains are comprised of 3 parts: reproductive structure, bran, and germ. If that sounds weird, simply bear with me for a second here. As I said, I'm supplying you with the nuts and bolts of the boring stuff so you'll understand the Paleo diet and have enough information to create a choice concerning whether or not it's the proper lifestyle for you. I feel everybody will have the benefit of eating Paleo, however, this is often ultimately one thing you've got to do for yourself and gauge however well you're feeling. Ok, back to grains:

Bran

Bran is that the outer covering of whole, unprocessed grain. It contains some vitamins, minerals, and a bunch of different proteins and anti-nutrients designed to forestall the predation or uptake of the grain.

Endosperm

The reproductive structure is starch with a touch little bit of protein. this is often the energy provider of a growing grain embryo.

Germ

The germ (sometimes cited as cereal germ) is that the portion of the grain that acts as its procreative system. In nature, the cereal grain is distributed by the wind, and once everything falls into place, the embryo begins the method of growth mistreatment the reproductive structure for energy. this is often the place where edible oil usually derives from.

A Note concerning Oats

I perceive that there are heaps of individuals out there who like to eat their morning oatmeal. however, I actually have some dangerous news... oatmeal contains many proteins kind of like protein. These proteins are laborious to digest, and so stay intact despite the simplest efforts of the digestive process to break them down. quite a bummer, right? Well, let me simply place it this way... attempt your best to travel with none form of grains for thirty days and see however you're feeling. I guarantee that you'll notice a significant distinction within the manner your digestive system, your energy levels, and your overall health and vitality work. I would like you to induce the term "whole grain" out of your head for the length of this experiment. this is often a term employed by the govt. to urge the US to assume that whole grains are a healthy substitute for natural foods.

A Word concerning Beans And Dairy

Several diets in today's diet world have incorporated the utilization of beans (or legumes) as a healthy substitute for carbohydrates and proteins at intervals your diet. Beans aren't essentially evil, however, they are doing results in similar issues as grains. Gut irritation, anti-nutrients, likewise as inflammation. I do eat black beans from time to time if I want I'm not obtaining enough carbs from my fruits and veggies.

Fats

Fats appears to be one amongst the foremost confusing aspects of the Paleo diet these days - and permanently reason. Ever since the office got concerned about the food processor, we've been told that fat could be a dangerous issue. this could be the reason however we've got to think about fat as a new price to every one meal we tend to eat. the overall population doesn't have a tough time understanding that carbs aren't smart for you. however once it involves fat, we are within the dark most the time. The funny issue concerning fat is our bodies are created of heaps of it. This includes our organs, brain, nerves, and even generative hormones. however, to accurately perceive however fat helps the body, you've got to grasp the subtypes of fats. There are 3 sorts of fats: saturated, monounsaturated, and unsaturated. You don't need to perceive everything concerning the science behind it, however, it's smart to grasp the fundamentals thus you're not within the dark.

Monounsaturated Fats

This type of fat is usually cited as monounsaturated fatty acid and is found in the main in foods like avocado, olive oil, and nuts (almonds, walnuts, etc.). however, this sort of fat is additionally found in grass-fed beef, which happens to be one amongst the staples of the Paleo diet. These fats are literally quite superb, as they have an inclination to assist improve insulin sensitivity, improve hormone response, and reduce sterol levels.

Polyunsaturated Fats

While monounsaturated fats are usually thought of as a healthier form of fat, unsaturated fatty acids are higher for you than saturated fatty acids. this is often as a result of being noted to scale back unhealthy cholesterol (LDL) and increase smart cholesterol (HDL). unsaturated fats additionally contain essential fatty acids like omega-3 and omega-6 fatty acid. These are fatty acids that the body wants, however, it cannot essentially turn out on its own. These sorts of fats also are vital because they send a symptom to your brain to allow you to apprehend after you are full. this may forestall bad eating habits and may additionally assist you to lose weight. The bottom line, unsaturated fats are vital.

Cut The Trans Fats!

Let's simply say that trans fats aren't the simplest issue for you. however, I'm positive you've detected others mention this. Trans fats are created once unsaturated fats from foods like corn and soybeans are exposed to heat. The resulting fats look kind of like saturated fats. they need a name for damaging the liver operation and destroying insulin sensitivity.

The Omegas (Omega-3 and Omega-6)

These sorts of fats are vital as they assist in dealing with inflammation within the body, and are famous to assist control numerous cancer components (typically in something that's associated with inflammation issues). omega-3 fatty acids are classified as an anti-inflammatory drug, whereas polyunsaturated fatty acid is classified as pro-inflammatory. The goal with our nutrition ought to be to even the ratio between these 2 Omegas. the general public is lacking in polyunsaturated fatty acid, which might be satisfied with foods like wild fish, grass-fed beef, and a few egg sources. polyunsaturated fatty acid also can be taken in supplement kind, however, attempt to minimize the utilization of supplements the maximum amount as attainable once making an attempt to stay to a Paleo diet.

List of polyunsaturated fatty acid Foods
You Should Be Eating:
•Wild salmon
•Anchovies
•Mackerel
•Herring
•Trout
•Omega-3 Eggs
•Grass-Fed Natural Beef
•An assortment of nuts and seeds (walnuts and linseed, for example)

CHAPTER 6

The Transformative Logic of the Paleo Diet

The underlying logic upon that the Paleo Diet is predicated on the idea that the genetic composition of recent man has been programmed towards the diet of our stone-age forefathers and it's not modified since. For quite 2.5 million years, man has had a similar natural diet consisting of untamed plants and animals such a lot that the shape has already become familiar with it. The human genetics is believed to be already programmed towards this sort of diet and also the agricultural and historic period within the last 10,000 years has not remodeled it. This can be the transformative logic on which the Paleo Diet relies.

The premise states that the biological science of recent man had scarcely modified through these years even once the arrival of modern agriculture and animal farming and despite the big scale modernization of food handling. They believe the 10,000 years covering the time once man initially learned in what way to cultivate plants and domesticate animals up to now when the trendy urban diet evolved wasn't enough to reprogram human genetics. Besides, modern humans started following the fashionable urban diet consisting mostly of processed food barely two hundred years past such that it'd be not possible for the body to entirely reprogram what took it 2.5 million years to program. Worst, the body is reacting negatively to the trendy urban diet as manifested through numerous chronic diseases that currently plague humans.

It was a gastroenterologist by the name of Walter L. Voegtlin who initially toyed with the construct of the stone-age diet someday within the mid-70's. Since then, a variety of books and tutorial journals are written regarding it. Together, they show that there's increasing proof to prove that a diet consisting of lean meat, fish, fruit, and vegetables just like the diet of our prehistoric ancestors will stop the alleged diseases of wealth trendy men are currently usually afflicted with.

The Paleo diet grew in quality and as its acceptance was simply obtaining a kickstart, some authors and scientists tried to introduce some modifications to the current construct confusing some advocates within the method. Others questioned the validity of its therefore known as transformative logic while not providing proof to negate the construct. Never-the-less, the Paleo diet still captured the imagination of a growing range of health and fitness advocates and it currently seems it's here to remain.

Followers of the Paleo Diet believe that to make sure health and well being, and stay free from diseases of richness, Homo sapiens must adapt to a diet that resembles the diet of his prehistoric ancestors. This transformative logic of the Paleo construct didn't sit well with some quarters. A variety of dieticians and anthropologists, particularly people who champion alternative modern-day dietary programs have questioned its validity claiming that an abundant of the Paleo construct is simply supported guesswork.

True enough, all of the health professionals who championed the Paleo Diet support like Walter L. Voegtlin and Dr. Lorain Cordain didn't live nonetheless throughout the Paleolithic era to be able to have a primary account of what the prehistoric individuals had for his or her meals. primarily, we will say that almost all of the contentions they wrote regarding were mere suppositions. However, in spite of however presumptive the Paleo construct is, it's not entirely unsupported.

The truth is the way of the Paleo assumptions were culled from well-documented studies and in-depth laboratory analyses that embody thorough analysis of the dental perform morphology of Hominin Fossil Records and Paleoenvironmental modeling among others. The principles are scientifically sound, the logic extremely affordable.

We don't seem to be but, about to take into a lot of bookish aspects of the primal diet. What we tend to are more fascinated by whether or not following the diet above can facilitate people to stay healthy and free from the direful diseases and diseases that are joined to the fashionable urban diet. For us, we will provide no higher proof than the varied up to date hunter-gatherer tribes still existing nowadays in various components of the world who still live on an identical primal diet. there's the Hazda Tribe of Tanzania, the Veddas of Sri Lanka, and also the Mbuti pygmies in Congo, the Guyana Indians of the Republic of Paraguay, the Eskimos of Alaska, the Aborigines of Australia, and also the East Coast yank Indians. The chronic diseases of affluence Homo sapiens are at risk of are much absent among these tribes. they're the proof positive of how primal diet is very important to keep the shape healthy and illness free. If you would like a lot of scientific basis showing the efficaciousness of the Paleo Diet, here's one incontrovertible proof for you which of them Paleo detractors attempt to merely ignore as a result of they can not contradict it.

Researchers from the University of American state San Francisco (UCSF) headed by Dr. Timothy White and Dr. Linda Frasseto did an actual check on a bunch of individuals who were all thought-about as unhealthy or have a disorder of some type. The subject was given a Paleo Diet consisting of lean meat, contemporary fruits, fish, nuts, and vegetables. after simply two weeks on this diet, the pressure level of everybody within the group went down dramatically, whereas steroid alcohol and glyceride levels born a median of thirty points – a feat that in line with Dr. Frasseto would have taken medicine like lipid-lowering medicine and alternative cholesterol-lowering medications six months to attain.

There are uncounted alternative stories of however the Paleo diet helped unwell people regain their health several of that were never printed. innumerable accounts of how the diet helped improve the physique and therefore the the} performance of skilled athletes also abound. The diet isn't a mere fad as the majority are created to believe by its detractors. it's a lifestyle. in truth it's well on its thanks to changing into the lifestyle of the longer term – the exact reason why proponents of alternative dietary regiments {try to|attempt to|try and} discredit its real price by tagging it as a non-civilized approach of uptake and living. sadly, they need however to contradict its effectiveness that several of its advocates would swear to even with their own lives.

CHAPTER 7

Your Paleo searching List

It would be too oversimplified to mention that the Paleo diet consists of lean meat from grass-fed, free-ranging placental and organically big fruits and vegetables. However, this might be imprecise for people that are making an attempt at the Paleo for the primary time, therefore, we need to prepare a Paleo shopping list to guide you on what to shop for the future time you shopping for food.

Lean Meat

Your main supply of proteins ought to be from the lean meat of naturally raised animals. Being naturally raised means that they were grass fed (not grain or corn fed) and are endocrine and antibiotic free. consistent with executive department standards, lean cuts of meat ought to contain solely a complete of five grams of fat, no quite a pair of grams of saturated fat, and solely ninety-five milligrams of cholesterin per 3.5 ounces of serving.

They should be cut off all visible fat and cartilage the maximum amount as doable. you'll be able to eat the maximum amount of those meats as you wish and for as long as you follow these preparation tips:

Make sure you drain off all the surplus fat. never deep fry meat to keep else fat to the minimum. Instead, attempt cookery, baking, or preparation. If you'll sauté any of them try and use as very little else oil as doable. Limit consumption of animal organs to eighty-five grams a month.

The following are the suggested lean meat sources and therefore the selection cuts:

Buffalo or bovid meat (any cut), Beef (flank cut, prime cut of meat, bottom or top round, eye of spherical, and alternative lean cuts, beef ought to be ninetieth lean), Chicken (skinless breast meat, additional lean ground chicken meat), Turkey (skinless white turkey meat and additional lean ground turkey meat), Duck, Goat (any cut), Pork (Bone-in rib chop, bone-in cut of meat roast, tenderloin, boneless high loin chop and roast, center loin, ground pork that's ninetieth lean), Lamb (arm, leg, and loin, shank, ground meat should be ninetieth lean), Eggs from non-poultry raised chickens, Animal organs from the afore listed animals like kidneys, bone marrow, liver, tongue, and sweet bread, Game meats like rabbit, wild boar, or cervid (any cut).

FISH

The micronutrients found in fish are found to spice up brain power and development. Fish ought to, therefore, be a part of your everyday Paleo diet meals whenever attainable. Fish and alternative food are glorious sources of macromolecule and Omega three. keep in mind tho' to forever select fish caught within the wild over farmed fish. Avoid canned fish too. in contrast to meat, the fattier fish are additional nutrient since they contain more useful fats and alternative micronutrients and Vitamins A, C, and E. The supplementary common wild-caught fish you may notice within the market are: Salmon

TUNA
Other ocean foods include Shellfish like shrimp, crab, lobsters, clams, mussels, and scallops.

FRUITS

There aren't any restrictions for fruits within the Paleo diet. you'll be able to eat any fruit that you like and consume the maximum amount as you want. However, if you're attempting to lose some pounds, it's best to limit the consumption of dates, mangoes, bananas, watermelon, and pineapple. they need the most sugar content and it's best to consume them sparsely. Dried fruits need to be avoided as they're jam-choked with sugar. Eat more avocados due to the reason that they contain a load of healthy fats.

VEGETABLES

All nonstarchy vegetables just like the dark leaved greens, pumpkins, herbs, and seaweeds are allowed within the Paleo diet. Starchy tubers like potatoes and legumes

NUTS AND SEEDS

Raw, unseasoned dried fruits and seeds are a part of Paleo snacks. The list includes cashews, almonds, pistachios, Brazil and pine nuts, pumpkin seeds, flower seeds, herb seeds, flaxseeds, and pumpkin seeds.

OILS

Avoid utilizing oil, groundnut oil or oil for preparation. they're extremely refined oils and per se have higher concentrations of inflammation inflicting unsaturated polyunsaturated fatty acid fats than the inflammation reducing omega three fats. Use instead the following: Virgin copra oil for every type of preparation Avocado oil for sauce or for low heat cooking vegetable oil for any quite cooking and as salad dressing too vegetable oil for seasoning and low heat cooking walnut oil for seasoning flaxseed oil not for cooking or seasoning except for direct intake as omega three supplement. the utilization of those Paleo counseled oils can facilitate maintain the balance between the omega three and omega half dozen fatty acids in our body.

Paleo Beverages

Soda and alternative bottled beverages are out of the list. This includes bottled or canned fruit juices that are ordinarily high in targeted sugar. Below are the counseled Paleo friendly beverages that can be used but without adding any extra sweeteners.

Coconut Water

Drink sugarless coconut milk and resultantly it'll have various health advantages like antioxidant properties, it's advantages against polygenic disease, it provides you higher viscus health, keeps you hydrated and prevents urinary organ stones.

Coffee

Drink black coffee or espresso, however, don't drink any lattes or sweet coffees as they're going to drive you far from your paleo lifestyle.

PALEO TREATS and SWEETS

The Paleo lifestyle isn't all that uninteresting and drab. there's an area for infrequent alcohol as long as you don't make it in one drinking session. you will conjointly take pleasure in dark chocolates to your heart's delight. they're smart for the heart. If you're trying to find sweetener, use raw honey which is sold at the farmers market instead.

Making Sure Your Meat is Paleo

Ideally, Paleo meat should be from free-ranging live stocks and are grass fed instead of corn or grain fed. Not only are they better, however, but they're also conjointly healthier and a lot more delicious. those who have tasted free travel chicken would swear to the current reality. Meat from herd animals that touched freely on pasture lands, and pigs and chickens set free on the sector are more delicious and quite a lot more nourishing. The primary ever staple food of our prehistoric ancestors is meat from wild animals they were able to seek out.

Paleo is regarding reversing the ill-effects of an excessive industrial enterprise to our lives that have conjointly modified our consumption habits dramatically. It's regarding consuming a lot more natural and organic food just like the cavemen did countless years past and therefore the meat was one among their 1st staple foods. just like the meat of our ancestors, the meat meant for inclusion in Paleo diets should be from a pasture-raised farm animal. Please observe that there's a giant distinction between pasture finished farm animal and the ones that are entirely grass-fed throughout their existence. Most of the pasture finished cows spent the primary half their lives subsisting on grain fed diets and were allowed solely to cast the pasture to kill grass only before they're sent to the butchery. they're not entirely freed from antibiotics and artificial food supplements.

Buy solely AGA certified grass-fed meat. AGA stands for the American Grassfed Association. American Grassfed Association meat merchandise certification is a time they were weaned up to the time they were harvested. The association was a guarantee that the merchandise came from farm animals fed solely with grass from the pastures and was founded in 2003 by organic livestock producers, veterinarians, and a grazing range management specialists to push the grass-fed business. they need producer-members in almost every state and their merchandise is sold-out in supermarkets similarly to numerous farmers markets inside the immediate vicinities of their farms. you must not have a problem finding American Grassfed Association certified meat merchandise within the country. you will even order meat merchandise online from a number of these producers. For additional info on American Grassfed Association producers. purchase game meat whenever and where ever attainable. the simplest meat that approximates the sort of meat ingested by our Paleo ancestors is game meat. This includes rabbit, deer, buffalo, ostrich, and swine thriving within the wild. they're not tough to get as there are brick and mortar outlets furthermore as on-line shops wherever you'll be able to purchase game meat. they probably will be priced more than the regular meat sold in supermarkets however they're a lot more delicious, similarly exotic and healthier. There are restaurants too that feature exotic game meats in their menus.

Don't obtain farmed fish and ocean food. Farmed fish are those that are farmed in massive scales like shrimps, tilapia, salmon, and milkfish. Farmed fish and food don't get to eat their natural food. they're given an organic from grains instead. Farmed fish have sometimes high mercury content. confirm the fish or food you purchase isn't farmed however caught from the ocean, lake, or ocean and not industrially farmed on an oversized scale. how would you know? Inquire! Ask the seller where the fish or ocean food came from.

Don't obtain chicken and alternative poultry merchandise that was raised on a commercial scale. the likelihood is that they're grain fed. hunt for free-ranging chickens. Don't assume they're onerous to search out. you'll be able to even shop for organically adult, free-ranging chickens in supermarkets however your best bet would be the farmer's markets. There are online sources too and possibly, identical sources wherever you purchase your lean meat additionally carry free-ranging chickens available for sale.

The Paleo guide to selecting chicken

The Free-range Chickens

The free-ranging chickens, on the opposite hand, are continuously loose to freely go outdoors. they're allowed to kill plants and insects. They feed freely on their scrounging for food in their natural environment and allowed to grow on its own with no growth-boosting hormones or nourishment supplements. they're conjointly organic.

The Organic Chickens

The organic chickens are chickens raised in giant numbers in a very wide, contained and controlled the atmosphere wherever they're allowed to additionally kill insects and plants. they're given solely natural organic feeds like vegetables however sans grain-based industrial feeds. Their atmosphere is herbicide, fungicide, and chemical free. they're conjointly not given antibiotics or growth-boosting hormones.

Chicken's nutritionary advantages:

The chicken meat has low sterol and fats but it is abundant in supermolecule and loaded with vitamins and minerals like vitamin B complex that is known to spice up the beneficial cholesterol (HDL) in your body, vitamin B complex that helps convert carbohydrates into fuel, element that are best-known inhibitors, an element that is required by the body for correct cell functions. Chicken meat is additionally a decent supply of supermolecule. Here may be a note of concern for you. If you don't wish to induce traces of harmful chemicals further from pesticides, fungicides, herbicides, and artificial food supplements and business feeds, it'll do the best for you to remain organic and stick with the Paleo food list.

The industrial Chickens

The business chickens are raised in giant scales in overcrowded poultries or cages often sprayed with pesticides, fungicides, and herbicides. they're fed with grain-based business feeds and their growth is increased with hormones and victuals supplements whereas their health is fortified with antibiotics to protect against pestilence and sickness.

Paleo Extreme: consuming Raw Food

People usually asked if Paleo is the caveman's diet then shouldn't consuming raw food be an integral part of it. the fact is that the Paleo diet encourages the consumption of food in their most state of nature as attainable. feeding raw food is, therefore, an important part of it. however, it's not such a lot as a result of our Paleolithic ancestors ate food that means but primarily because it brings important nutritionary advantages that should not be unnoticed. For one issue, raw food is live food. other than being wealthy in nutrients, it conjointly contains natural life energy. change of state food diminishes this life energy and destroys the nutrients considerably rendering it nutritiously useless. Doesn't it build a lot of sense to place living food into your body than food that has been rendered lifeless by cooking?

If the conception of live food and life energy appear unlikely to you, then at least take into account this. The food contains natural enzymes that facilitate break down the nutrients and aid the digestion and absorption of food. change of state destroys abundant of those enzymes. Of course, the body will manufacture these enzymes to assist within the digestion and absorption of the prepared food we tend to eat. however, it makes the bodywork tougher to supply enzymes when the body takes in prepared food and therefore the body will solely do most. On the opposite hand, the consumption of raw food saves the body from the difficulty of manufacturing these enzymes.

Cooking food at a hundred and twenty degrees Fahrenheit or higher destroys all the natural enzymes and far of the nutrients in them. consuming prepared food with abundant of the enzymes destroyed because of the change of state at high-temperature forces the body to supply these enzymes so unnecessarily adding stress to that. Raw food diet already contains these enzymes then it saves the body from this extra stress. well-liked raw food diets taken by most raw food converts incorporates raw and unprocessed fruits and vegetables, cracked and seeds, eggs, tuna dish from fish, Carpaccio from meat, non pasteurized and non-homogenized milk, cheese, and yogurt.

Raw food enthusiasts can swear that consuming raw food is an exceptional energy booster. They profess that it offers them a moment of energy recharge. They conjointly claim they get to sleep deeper when consuming raw food, thus, they have fewer hours of sleep than is generally needed. consequently, they continuously come to life feeling choked with energy all the time.

These are their claims however a lot of concrete advantages that may be gained from a raw food diet in line with nutritionists include:

Significant weight loss - since it's primarily a coffee fat, low carb diet, higher digestion owing to the natural enzymes within the diet, Regularity within the movement since the diet is high in fiber, Lessens the chance of getting heart diseases and different diseases coupled to trans-fat and saturated fats within the food we tend to eat, Less water retention as a result of the diet is low in metal which implies it aids in maintaining a perfect weight, Protects against cancer since it's effective in cancer-fighting phytochemicals.

Paleo Raw Food for Detoxing

There is another important profit that may be gained with a Paleo Raw Food Diet - it rids the body of accumulated toxins. Toxins are harmful wastes or free radicals that are residues ensuing from breaking down food. they'll accumulate within the body through the years and harm cells which can even result in cancer. The body is unable to utterly disembarrass itself of those harmful toxins and through the time they accumulate to a degree that they hamper cell functions and have an effect on energy production and ultimately result in the event of diseases like cancer. feeding fiber-rich raw food diet helps the body get eliminate these toxins. Raw food diet contains antioxidants that neutralize the cell-damaging free radicals. It cleanses our organic process systems and fortifies the system.

CHAPTER 8

Formulating a recent Paleo Diet set up

Now that you just have a lot of or less a clearer understanding of the Paleo Diet, you've got to feel extremely driven to be able to adapt it to your lifestyle. And like every different nutritionary program, you've got to own an idea to place it into action. You can't simply dive in and play it by ear because it can solely result in failure and dismay. designing your switch to the Paleo lifestyle can guarantee your success as well as enable you to watch your progress. there's no "one size fits all" Paleo diet set up. each set up is unambiguously tailored to suit the wants and requirements of people. begin with a 28-day plan to eat solely Paleo food.

Below are some tips you'll be able to follow in formulating your planned transition to the Paleo modus vivendi.

Step one – take your beginning date. structure your mind once you wish the shift to begin and be firm regarding it. Don't take too long as you will get sidetracked by different things which will cause you to lose interest in it. Remember, it's your health and longevity at stake here.

Step two – Encourage members of the family to hitch in ever-changing over to the Paleo diet so you, therefore, won't be all by your lonesome self. Besides, with different members of the family within the same diet, you'd be able to inspire and facilitate one another out. it might be a fun and fulfilling journey the results of that are a few things everybody can care for for the remainder of their lives.

Step three – build a record of everything before you start on the program. Take measurements of yourself specifically your height and weight. See your doctor and have blood chemistry done on you to incorporate your blood sugars, CRP, pressure level, TG, HDL, LDL particle size, etc. All these can assist you to apprehend the sort of progress you're creating with the diet. And oh, don't forget to require an image of yourself with as very little garments on as doable. This may come in handy once examining you then and currently. write any health problems you will have before you begin on the diet. embody bloating, diarrhea, constipation, abdominal pain, acid reflux, gas, etc. this could complete the image of what you're before ever-changing over to the Paleo lifestyle.

Step four – free your room of all non-Paleo foodstuffs. Throw them away or to do better still, provide them intent on your neighbors. no matter you opt to try and do with them, make certain they're out of your sight and in a place wherever you can't be tempted to reach out for them.

Step five – go on a spree. Get your Paleo food list out and begin stocking up on them. Visit your friendly neighborhood foodstuff or grocery and if you can't notice some Paleo foodstuff there visit the farmers market. compose what you can't get from your nearest neighborhood food retailers and get them organized from on-line sources. The vital issue is to own everything Paleo in your room so you won't be tempted to use substitutes.

Step six – begin grouping Paleo Recipes and build a weekly design to last consecutive 28-day challenge. This way, you won't be at a loss on what to cook next.

Step seven – Don't take anybody weight measurements until after the twenty-eight days. however fastidiously compose any physical or emotional changes you will feel within the course of the challenge. this manner you won't get frustrated if the changes are slow in returning. Don't worry, the changes can happen.

Step eight – in spite of what happens or no matter it's you are feeling stick with your set up till the last day of the 28-day challenge. At the top of the 28-day challenge, fastidiously measure the progress you've created if any. it's the time to seek out if the Paleo diet created you healthier, feel higher, change state, or if it worsened your condition instead.

Evaluate by:

Taking another image of yourself sporting constant garments once you took the primary picture. you'll be able to currently visually compare if there are variations between then and now. Take your body measurements over again and compare your weight and your region then and currently. Get another blood chemistry work done and raise your doctor's facilitate to interpret and compare the results then and currently. There will solely be one reason why the challenge won't bring the expected results. It should be as a result of you're not serious enough to strictly pursue the challenge to its completion and somewhere on the road, you've indulged in some exceptions or bust the diet from time to time.

If you don't notice any enhancements for currently, maybe your body wants longer to adapt to the new diet, therefore, stick with the diet a touch longer till there are manifest results. If you've achieved nice progress, then it's up to you to determine whether or not you ought to stick with the Paleo diet permanently.

Below may be a sample weekly Paleo design. You shouldn't have any problem with fashioning a weekly Paleo design. begin by grouping as many Paleo recipes as you'll be able to and selected people whom you fancy most. Incorporate them into a weekly design ensuring there's selection, therefore, you won't get bored consuming identical stuff over and over again. There are a lot of free on-line sources for Paleo diet recipes.

CHAPTER 9

Modern Paleo Principles

The modern Paleo diet is constructed upon the assumption that man's health and well being is maintained by intense a diet consisting of slightly processed food that was obtainable before the arrival of agriculture.
There are but no set of mounted rules very similar to commandments written on stone. everyone seems to be too liberal to eat the maximum amount as he desires as long as what he consumes belong to the Paleo food list as delineate within the previous chapters. There aren't any zones to follow, neither are there calories to count.

To a lot of avid Paleo advocates, the diet is straightforward enough to follow except for the primary time converts, the absence of set rules is confusing and should even tempt them to form excuses certainly exemptions currently then and break the diet to splurge on certain indulgences. For the inexperienced, we've listed below some pointers or recommendations on what to try to and what to not do. they're by no means that a group of rules to follow however a set of recommendations to guide you through your 1st Paleo journey.

Wheat, rice, corn, and all alternative grains don't have any place within the Paleo diet. they're no better than a sweetener.

Junk foods and restaurant food ready with edible fat and artificial food supplements also are out. you must eat real food instead.

Refined sugar, syrup, corn syrup, and artificial sweeteners are out.

Virgin coconut oil, nut oil, and vegetable oil along with side animal fats like butter, tallow, ghee, and lard are in. Refined oils like oil, edible fat, corn oil, and soy oil are out. change fats are out still.

Beans, legumes, peanuts, tubers, farm merchandise, don't have any place within the Paleo diet too.

Paleo is over a diet. it's a way of life which implies other than food, movement within the style of exercises and rest by the manner of sleeping are even as necessary. Together, food, sleep, and movement represent the 3 foundations of the fashionable Paleo lifestyle. Short, high-intensity daily exercises can have the best for the desired movement.

You should additionally make certain you get enough sleep a day. provide your body enough time to recover when every physical exertion. never abuse your body the least bit.

Avoid contact chemically the maximum amount as potential. Don't drink H2O. it's extremely chlorinated or fluoridated. Drink drinking water instead. With similar logic, avoid swimming in chlorinated pools.

Use solely deodorants that are freed from aluminum, halide-free dentifrice, and a lot of natural organic soap.

Do some intermittent abstinence 2 or 3 times per week. you'll skip breakfast and morning occasional. you may skip lunch too if you prefer. By fasting, you're starving the body cells to induce them to allocate the nutrients from cells that don't seem to be functioning optimally to be used to fuel alternative cell functions. you must not try this a day tho' because the body can learn to adapt to that negating the aim of abstinence.

You can save a great deal if you be a part of Community-supported agriculture programs. There should be one in your neighborhood or anyplace close to you. they're the most affordable supply of contemporary Paleo foodstuff. contemplate shopping for food in bulk like buying half a cow, or a bovid, or maybe a lamb rather than shopping for by the pound. you may save a great deal more this way. Besides, you may get all the prime cuts too. you may want a deep-freeze tho' for this and begin learning the way to cook shanks, shoulders, tails, trotters, and hocks. you may have been avoiding them within the past in favor of the prime cuts however you may be stunned at however delicious they taste. On prime of that, they sell cheaper that's why they're referred to as thrift cuts. you may save a large amount of cash together with them in your hotel plan.

Make it some extent to go to the farmer's market close to the top of the day and not an hour earlier. The farmers would need to urge eliminate their merchandise before the day ends and are seeking to sell their turn out at a cut-price to anyone still hanging around the place instead of leaving them to waste.

Get organized. make certain you have got a Paleo searching list a weekly Paleo hotel plan. Check if all the Paleo ingredients for your weekly hotel plan are available. Being organizes from searching to change of state gets things done quicker and easier. you may additionally avoid shopping for too several things on impulse.

Make a minimum of a single day during a week your "Fish Day." On today eat solely no cooked fish like tuna fish salad with kippers for snacks with a great deal of raw inexperienced ivy-covered vegetables build use a great deal a part of your change of state. as an example, if you grill breast chicken these days, don't throw away the leftover. Store them within the white goods and use them for salad or fricassee every day or 2 later.

Don't be afraid to experiment change of state your meal from your Paleo instruction. try and produce one thing which will cause you to feel nice. There aren't any quick rules concerning making ready a Paleo meal as long as you keep on with the utilization of the Paleo food list. try and discover your vary of Paleo foods that cause you to feel nice and stick to it. Once again, don't be discouraged if you don't expertise immediate results. There are folks whose bodies want longer to regulate to a replacement diet. And don't be afraid if initially, you're feeling foggy or energetic. this can be a standard reaction once the body changes over to victimization fat for energy instead of from carbohydrates.

CHAPTER 10

Paleo Diet for Athletes

It is not solely those that have issues with their weight, or those searching for a cure for a few upset or unwellness who find the Paleo Diet healthfully useful. Even the able athletes within the peak of their form have found the Paleo to be the proper diet for them significantly the endurance athletes who usually pay several hours every day in intense coaching.

For years currently, biological process specialists are attempting to seem for that excellent food combination which will facilitate boost the athletes' endurance throughout coaching and guarantee wonderful performance during competitions. The biological process demand of the normal person who lives an inactive lifestyle is most a lot of differently from an athlete who is usually subjected to intense exertions virtually daily.

The Paleo diet seems to be a God-given gift to those champion athletes as most of them would attest to that. With the fashionable urban diet containing stuff that proves to be prohibitory to competitory athletes, nutritionists are scrambling to place along with a diet that's tailor-fitted to their specific biological process wants. As a result of that athletes bear intense workouts daily, Eat properly before, during, and when each physical exertion still as in between workouts is of overriding importance to confirm they need enough energy to realize peak performance and at a similar time facilitate their bodies recover quickly from the toilsome Exercise. the most focus of a perfect athlete's diet is to supply him with enough fuel to sustain him through several hours of intense energy output and to provide him nourishment when every session to assist the body recover quickly.

The ideal diet for endurance athletes should, therefore, be ready to do one issue - to keep up adequate glycemic masses within the blood the least bit times throughout the physical exertion. this could mean increasing saccharide consumption a lot of usually and in larger quantities than the traditional demand of the standard individual. Endurance athletes got to have a moderate intake of carbohydrates 2 hours before every intense physical exertion. this can provide the body enough time to bring the blood glucose to the suitable levels suited to rigorous exertions that need intense energy output. If the workouts are aiming to be tedious, the athlete might need to increase his saccharide intake often throughout the length of the exercise. For workouts that last no over an hour, water often would satisfy.

He should additionally eat foods wealthy in carbohydrates and with a modest quantity of supermolecule at intervals the primary 30 minutes when every physical exertion. this can be essential for quick and effective recovery. If necessary, he will continue intense high saccharide foods for many hours for an extended recovery. After this, he should return to his regular Paleo diet program. The nutrient demand of an athlete might vary from time to time looking at his coaching schedule. The saccharide and fat intake as shown described above schedule is meant to travel on well with the opposing swings in the athlete's energy utilization because the coaching progresses from totally different stages. it's vital to notice down these energy swings and program the saccharide and supermolecule intake consequently.

The Paleo Diet is, of course, Ergogenic maybe the foremost important feature of the Paleo Diet that specifically edges athletes is it being ergogenic. It means that it's packed with nutrients that enhance the performance of athletes. it's significantly high in animal supermolecule that is that the best supply of branched-chain amino acids like essential amino acid, valine, an essential amino acid that is liable for muscle growth and repair. the fashionable urban diet is often acidic and therefore the body's natural reaction to neutralize acidity by breaking down muscle tissues. Athletes on a Western diet unremarkably would realize it hard to keep up and enhance their muscle stores when a tough day's physical exertion. On the opposite hand, athletes on the Paleo Diet don't suffer supermolecule breakdown in their muscle mass. The Paleo diet produces a net alkalic result within the body that is that the actual opposite of what the up to date Western diet produces. This eliminates the requirement for the supermolecule-breaking reaction of the body to acidic diets, therefore, no protein muscle breakdown happens. The Paleo Diet for athletes needs to be changed to'. It should be tailored specifically to an athlete's coaching program and nutrient needs. It should be changed in such a manner that permits a tiny low window of chance for the consumption of starches and straightforward sugars by the athletes from non-Paleo sources throughout, before, and after the particular exercise. It should allow high carbo intake by athletes as required and once it suits them best whereas coaching each to stay them in their peak forms throughout the physical exertion session and to provide them the much-needed nutrients for his or her bodies to recover quickly in time for subsequent arduous exercise.

Outside of the coaching schedule, it's strictly Paleo all the manner – low carb, high supermolecule diet. which means intense loads of lean meat, seafood, poultry, vegetables, and contemporary fruits as much because the athletes like. To summarize, the Paleo Diet has the subsequent useful benefits for athletes as Compared to alternative diets accessible nowadays for endurance athletes:

The Paleo diet for athletes has a lot of the open chain amino acids which boosts muscle growth and anabolic perform. The Branched-chain amino acids conjointly stop or minimize the suppression of the system that ordinarily follows intensive workouts by endurance athletes.

The diet strikes a balance between the inflammation inflicting omega6 fatty acids and useful omega3 fatty acids. It reduces if not eliminates post-workout tissue inflammations that usually affect athletes once a strenuous physical exercise. The Paleo diet produces an alkalic result that lowers the body's acidity so reducing the debilitating effect of pathology on the bones and muscles whereas at a similar time causing supermolecule synthesis within the muscle tissues for a lot of muscle growth. The Paleo Diet includes nutrient-rich vegetables and food. they're filled with essential vitamins and trace minerals required by endurance athletes to take care of optimum health and for effective future recovery from hard exercises.

Training for such endurance sports as running, weight lifting, cycling, swimming, triathlon, rowing, and race marathons is onerous to the body. The endurance athlete is consistently in some variety of a recovery stage following each strenuous physical exercise. this can be wherever the Paleo diet is important to an athlete because it re-nourishes the body with the much-needed carbohydrates and proteins it lost within the coaching whereas at a similar time providing the body with trace nutrients and vitamins required to repair the body back to type. Together, the Paleo diet and a very quiet sleep become the essential elements of the endurance athlete's educational program.

The athlete must recover quickly and effectively once every serious physical exercise for him to be prepared and ready for succeeding. This has invariably been the largest challenge an endurance athlete faces in preparation for a contest. Let the reality be told, it'll be not possible for an athlete to form a full and quick recovery with a strictly all Paleo diet. What he consumes ought to be ready to make full the stored nutrients and polyose he lost on every coaching session and an occasional carb high supermolecule diet just like the Paleo diet won't fulfill as it is. that's why the Paleo diet must be changed to incorporate the employment of non-Paleo high sugar sources throughout, prior, and post-training. it's the sole way to guarantee speedy recovery in time for succeeding serious calculate. In short, a changed Paleo diet for jocks must be developed to accommodate all the nutrient needs of an endurance athlete.

Formulating the Paleo Diet for Athletes

As has been realized earlier, the Paleo diet must be slightly changed to suit the necessities of endurance athletes on coaching. Specifically, they have to enhance their sugar intake at totally different stages of every serious physical exercise. Before the physical exercise, sugar intake is required to boost the sugar load within the blood to a suitable level for the expected intense energy output. High sugar intake throughout the course of the physical exercise is additionally necessary to take care of peak performance. And to be ready to recover quickly from the hard physical exercise, sugar intake is once more required within the initial few hours in real time following the physical exercise to assist the body recover quickly and be prepared for succeeding. Again, the modifications ought to be slight and temporary long enough to last the length of the coaching period. There are not any quick and firm rules on however one ought to move it. It shouldn't, however, veer away too far away from the fundamental Paleo ideas.

Below are some basic Paleo Principles you'll be able to use in customizing your Paleo diet for athletes:

Leave out all processed foods from your food list and eat solely natural organic foods. Processed foods have artificial ingredients that will impact your body chemistry and have an effect on your performance furthermore as your health.

Make fruits and vegetables, haywire and seeds, as your main supply of carbohydrates. Limit your consumption of sugary energy drink supplements to coaching sessions. Take them solely as required however avoid them for the remainder of the day.

20 to 25th of your calorie demand should be from animal supermolecule significantly from grass-fed farm animal and poultry, game meats and from non-farmed fish and food.

Increase your consumption of fish and walnuts and alternative sources of omega- three fatty acids to balance the presence of inflammation inflicting omega six from other food sources.

Don't eat food cooked with trans fat like canola, corn, and soy oil. If you wish to fry food use vegetable oil or virgin oil instead. It is much better to don't fry, grill or broil instead. Processed snack foods are high in trans fats, therefore, avoid them too. you furthermore might need to limit your consumption of saturated fats.

Leave out all dairy farm merchandise from your diet.

Drink an abundance of water. keep it your main fluid intake.

Other a lot of specific modifications on the Paleo diet for athletes can depend upon the character of the game, the volume, and intensity of the coaching furthermore as on the physical build of the athlete. Generally, the larger the athlete is, or the tougher or longer the coaching, a lot of carbohydrates are required - before, during, and after the physical exercise.

Power athletes like sprinters, weight lifters, football players, and swimmers, as an example, need to consume one gram of supermolecule per pound of weight during a day as a general rule. Others have benefited enormously from what Doctor Mauro Di- Pasquale calls a 'cyclical low sugar diet' wherever they get to consume higher carbohydrate intake once or double per week solely to condition the body to burn fat for fuel too. Dr. Di-Pasquale could be a recognized authority on dietary regimens for athletes.

CHAPTER 11

PALEO RECIPES

PALEO BRAKFAST RECIPES

FROM THE GARDEN BASIL CHICKEN SALAD

Ingredients:

2 enormous destroyed, and pre-cooked skinless chicken bosoms

2 little pittedavocadoes

1/3 cup de-stemmed basil leaves

2 ½ tbsp. olive oil

¼ tsp. dark pepper

¼ tsp. ocean salt

Directions:

Start by situating the destroyed chicken in your blending bowl.Next, include the olive oil, the avocado, the basil, the salt, and the pepper to a food processor. Heartbeat the fixings until they're totally smooth.Add this blend over the destroyed chicken and hurl the chicken well to coat it completely. Season the chicken to taste, and enable it to rest in the refrigerator prior to serving.

CHINESE-BASED CABBAGE CHICKEN SALAD

Ingredients:

1 ¾ cup hacked and cooked chicken
4 cups chopped savoy cabbage 1/3 cup
1/3 cup julienned scallions
1 cup julienned carrot
1/3 cup hacked cilantro
1/3 cup julienned radishes 1/3 cup hacked mint

Dressing Ingredients:

2 tbsp. sesame oil
2 ¼ tbsp. coconut vinegar
2 ½ tbsp. coconut aminos
1 diced chipotle pepper
juice from ½ lime
1 tsp. nectar
3 minced garlic cloves
1 tsp. diced ginger

Directions:

Start by combining the hacked and julienned carrots, cabbage, scallions, what's more, radishes. Include the mint, the cilantro, and the slashed chicken, and hurl the plate of mixed greens in an enormous blending bowl. Next, position the serving of mixed greens to the side. To make the vinaigrette, start by expelling the chipotle pepper seeds. Spread the pepper with water and enable it to sit for thirty minutes.

Following thirty minutes, add the pepper to the sustenance processor and heartbeat it for one minute before adding different fixings to the processor. Taste the vinaigrette what's more, change the flavors, in the event that you please. Pour the dressing over the made serving of mixed greens, and prepare the plate of mixed greens to coat.

MEXICAN-INSPIRED CHICKEN TACO SALAD

Ingredients:

2 tbsp. taco flavoring (made beneath)
½ pound destroyed chicken
1/3 cup water
1 tbsp. olive oil
1 head destroyed lettuce
1 diced tomato
1 diced red onion
1 little, hollowed avocado
½ diced green pepper

Directions:

Start by combining the taco flavoring, as followings.
Unite 1 tsp. garlic powder, 4 tbsp. bean stew powder, 2 tsp. paprika 1 tsp. onion powder 1 tsp. oregano, ¼ tsp. red pepper pieces, 3 tsp. salt Blend the fixings before taking out the 2 tbsp. of the taco flavoring you require for this formula. (Note that you can keep the flavoring for a later formula, if you so pick.) Next, heat the olive oil in the skillet. Add the chicken to the olive oil to give it an increase in flavor. Pour the water overtop, alongside the taco flavoring. Enable the chicken blend to stew until the water totally vanishes. Next, cut up the various fixings. Make the serving of mixed greens by amassing together the vegetables, the chicken, and so forth. Hurl the fixings well, and appreciate!

AVOCADO-BASED PALEO CHICKEN SALAD

Ingridients:

3 skinless and boneless chicken bosoms, pre-cooked and destroyed
1/3 diced onion
1 diced avocado
2 tbsp. lime juice
3 tbsp. cilantro
salt and pepper to taste

Directions:

Bring all the above fixings together and blend well, making a point to crush the avocado as you go. Enjoy this exceptionally straightforward formula.

Muffins made up of Almond Flour

Ingredients:

1 cup blanched almond flour (4 oz)
two eggs
one tbsp century plant nectar or honey
¼ tsp hydrogen carbonate
½ tsp apple vinegar

Instructions:

Combine almond flour and hydrogen carbonate in an exceedingly medium-size bowl. combine the eggs, agave, and vinegar in an exceedingly larger bowl Cut within the dry ingredients into the egg mixture, mix well till the material is consistent. Scoop batter into a paper lined quick bread pan ¼ cup at a time. Heat kitchen appliance to 350° and bake muffins for quarter-hour or till the perimeters are slightly tanned Cool the muffins whereas still within the pan for a minimum of half an hour. Add butter and raspberry jam

Makes four muffins. You can use identical ingredients and therefore the same directions to form a fast bread loaf. simply double the ingredients and bake it longer – forty to forty-five minutes rather than quarter-hour. Use a little loaf pan.

PALEO NUTTY BARS FOR BREAKFAST

Ingredients:

1 Cup almond flour (blanched)
¼ tsp kosher salt
two tbsp honey
¼ C copra oil, one tbsp water
½ Cup sliced coconut (unsweetened)
¼ C raisins
½ Cup pumpkin seeds
¼ Cup almonds (blanched slivered
one tsp seasoning
½ Cup flower seeds

Instructions:

Combine and blend salt and almond flour in a baking oven. Cut in water, honey, copra oil, and vanilla. Add cut coconut, almond slivers, raisins, pumpkin seeds, and flower seeds.
Place the dough firmly into a regular baking pan, and pat down the dough utilizing your hands wet with water. Bake for twenty minutes at 350°.

PALEO PORRIDGE

Ingredients:

two mashed bananas
a pair of Cup coconut milk
1/4 Cup flax meal
3/4 Cup almond meal
one tsp cinnamon
1/8 tsp ground cloves
1/2 tsp ginger
1/8 tsp ground nutmeg
syrup or raw honey as sweetener
1/8 tsp coarse ocean salt
You may add unsweetened coconut flakes berries, nuts, or seeds, for topping.

Instructions:
Use a medium-size pan. place altogether the ingredients and simmer on low heat. Stir often till thick and produces bubbles. it'll be at the start skinny however will bite by bit thicken as you cook. it'll thicken therefore a lot of when cookery until up to serving time so it's best that you simply add a bit further coconut milk or water. high with berries or coconut flakes before serving.

KALE SALAD

Ingredients:

1 few kale leaves, three ounces Andouille sausage, 1/2 cup sliced mushrooms, ½ cup diced onion, one/4 cup + 1 tablespoon further virgin oil, a pair of tbsp apple vinegar, one tsp + a lot of to style, 1/2 tsp cracked black pepper, a pair of eggs deep-fried.

Instructions:
Slice the kale leaves by removing the stalks and dense spines. Rinse, and pat dry thoroughly. Dice the kale leaves into bite-sized pieces, put away in a big blender. Cut the Andouille sausage and cook on medium fire one tablespoon of the oil and a medium-sized frypan. Cook sausage till a lot of the fat has been taken out and consequently the sausage is somewhat crisp. Add the mushrooms and onions and simmer for five more minutes. Lower the heat and add a quarter cup of oil in conjunction with pepper, salt, and apple vinegar. Stir well for some seconds till everything is heated through. Pour the still hot Andouille sausage dressing over the kale and put away. Fry 2 eggs. Throw the dish with the dressing and divide among 2 plates. Serve the dish with the egg on top of it.

PALEO LUNCH RECIPES

Beef Barbacoa

Ingredients:

Six pounds small beef roast cuts

eight garlic cloves
six slices chiptole peppers
six peppers
one tbsp dried oregano
three tbsp coconut oil
two tbsp ground cumin
one tablespoon black pepper powder
five bay leaves
one tbsp Kosher salt
half cup of apple vinegar
six tablespoon of lime juice
1 teaspoon of cloves
ground 1 1/2 cups beef stock
two pieces of juniper berries.

Instructions:

Heat two tbsp of oil on a medium heat using a large pan. Pan Fry each side of the meat for about two to three minutes making sure they are cooked or properly browned. Place the lightly tanned meat in a Crockpot.
Put the vinegar, adobo sauce, chipotle peppers, garlic, oregano, lime juice, cumin, salt, black pepper, and cloves in a food blender and mix until it is smooth. Pour blended sauce over meat and then add the beef stock and then garnish the top of the meat.
Cover the crockpot and use a low flame to cook for six hours until the meat is very tender.
Transfer the liquid into a wide bottom pan and let simmer on high heat until the quantity is reduced by only one half of the original quantity.

Paleo Chicken Fajitas

Ingredients:

3 pounds sliced chicken breast piece
three sliced onions
three bell peppers
five garlic cloves(finely chopped)
lemon juice (four lemons)
three tablespoons each of oregano
cumin, coriander and chili powder
four tablespoons of coconut oil
lettuce leaves and butter for serving the fajitas
You have the choice for your fajita toppings. It can anything from chopped tomatoes, sliced avocados, pickles, guacamole, sauerkraut, and mayonnaise.

Instructions:

Blend the onions, chicken, bell peppers, garlic and spices in a blender. Mix them well inside the blender and put the mixture in the white sauce to infuse it for four hours, take a big enough fry pan and heat it under low flame and add the oil. Put the chicken that is marinated into the frypan and cook the bell peppers and onion are crisp and also the chicken is completely prepared. Now, transfer the chicken and veggies mixture into a large enough bowl and now to make a fajita with placing the lettuce leaves and top it any of the veggies garnish.

Garlic mussels with White Wine

Ingredients:

four lbs new mussels
two chopped onions
five finely hacked cloves garlic
two cups white wine or chicken stock
six tbsp spread or ghee
 1/3 cup of your preferred herbs.

Directions:

Wash the mussels altogether and clean its hair. Discard the majority of the opened mussels cooking. Utilize a stockpot for cooking. Spot the white wine, garlic and onions and heat to the point of boiling. Stew for around 5 minutes before including the cleaned mussels. Spread and raise the temperature to medium-high. Give it a chance to bubble until every one of the mussels is open. Include the herbs and spread (or ghee) before expelling the pot from the flame. Serve in dishes with margarine sauce, white wine, and garlic.

Pork slashes with apples and onions

Ingredients:
Four pork slashes bone-in and with trimmings
two enormous onion(sliced)
three tbsp crude margarine
four apples(cut with center removed)
Pepper and Salt.

Guidelines:

Rub the pork slashes with salt and pepper. Spot a huge dish on a stove over medium-high warmth and soften two tablespoons of your favored cooking fat. Sear each side of the pork hacks for five minutes or until caramelized and appropriately cooked. Put in a safe spot for some time. Set the warmth among medium and low at that point include the rest of the 1 tablespoon of fat. Include apple cuts and cut onions. Cook for at any rate four minutes or until the apple cuts are somewhat delicate and the onions have all the earmarks of being as of now caramelized. Top the pork slashes with cooked apple cuts and onions and serve.

Gluten-Free Chicken Strips

Ingredients:
1/2 lbs. boneless chicken chest parts
1 tbsp grapeseed oil

⅓ C coconut oil
½ cup coconut flour
¾ cup destroyed coconut
½ tsp salt
12 pounds crisp black pepper
1 egg

Guidelines:

Set the broiler temperature at 4000 F. While preheating the broiler, set up the flour blend. Consolidate flour with pepper and salt in a blending bowl (medium size). Beat the egg together with 1 tbsp of grapeseed oil in a different bowl. Spot the precut coconut in another bowl. Plunge the chicken pieces first in the flour blend ensuring each piece is covered equitably. Plunge the chicken pieces into the egg blend than on the destroyed coconut. Organize the covered chicken pieces in a low sided heating container and shower with coconut oil or softened spread. Heat for fifteen to twenty minutes turning the chicken over once.

Basic Shrimp Scampi

Ingredients:

1 lb of shrimp or prawns
3 tbsp field margarine or ghee
3 cloves of garlic (finely slashed)
1/2 lemon squeezed
Salt and Pepper

Guidelines:

Warm your griddle first before including the margarine. When the skillet is hot enough diminish the warmth to medium-low and include the margarine. Include the garlic once the margarine is dissolved. Include the recently washed and dried shrimps. Sauté the shrimps for 10 minutes or until they are never again translucent. Expel from the flame and include the lemon juice. Raced with some salt and pepper before serving hot.

Broiled Chicken with Citrus and Garlic

Indredients:

1 entire chicken
1 cup onion iodized salt
1 orange
Some water to cover the feathered creature in a stock pot
Roasting the Chicken
1 stick field spread
cut into 1 inch thick cuts

1 lemon
1 huge orange
3 sprigs rosemary finely chopped
6 cloves garlic finely chopped
Barely any drops of Extra Virgin Olive Oil

Guidelines:

Brining the Chicken

Evacuate the giblets and put the chicken in a huge stock pot and spread with water. Heat some water in a different container including one cup of salt until all the salt is broken up. Include the bubbled salted water together with the squeezed orange (incorporate the skin) to the huge stock pot with chicken and permit to marinate for at least 3 hours or maybe even close to 5 hours inside the fridge.

Broiling the Chicken

Preheat the stove to 425. Gently wash the marinated chicken and pat dry. With your fingers, make a 'spread pocket' by isolating the chicken skin from the bosoms. Spot the spread cuts to the 'margarine pockets' under the skin together with half of the hacked garlic.

Addition the oranges, lemons, the rest of the garlic and rosemary inside the chicken cavity. Leave some rosemary for embellishing. Brush the skin of the chicken with a little olive oil at that point sprinkle with the leftover rosemary. Cook the chicken at 425 degrees for 90 minutes. In the wake of broiling the chicken haul it out of the stove and brush the outside skin with liquefied margarine in the heating container. Cut and serve.

Paleo Chicken Salad Wraps

Ingredients:

1/2 cup cleaved cooked or bubbled chicken
3 tbsp cleaved Fuji apples
2 tbsp cleaved red grapes
2 tsp nectar
2 tbsp almond margarine

Guidelines:

Make a simple Paleo chicken serving of mixed greens by combining all fixings. Envelop the chicken plate of mixed greens by a Romaine leaf and serve.

Paleo Nutty Meatloaf Recipe

Ingridients:

1 lb ground meat

5 cloves garlic, minced
1 little green pepper finely hacked
1 tsp basil finely grounded
1 tsp rosemary finely grounded
1 tsp thyme finely grounded
½ cup of blended ground almonds, pecans, and walnuts
2 eggs
Black pepper, ground

Directions:

Put every one of the fixings in a major blending bowl. Make sure the fixings are uniformly joined in the blend. Spot the blend in the fridge for 30 minutes to 60 minutes. Oil a portion container utilizing olive oil and move the blend into it. Heat for one hour and 15 minutes. Cut and serve.

Paleo Steak with Mushroom and Onion Gravy

Ingredients:

3 pieces 6-ounce Sirloin steak
1 cup coconut milk
2 tbsp coconut flour
1 medium onion cut
2 to 3 garlic cloves squashed
1/8 tsp cayenne pepper
1/4 tsp ocean salt
1/2 cup cut mushrooms
1/2 tsp dark pepper
1 tbsp coconut oil

Directions:

Setting up the Steaks:

Sear, flame broil, or sauté the steak to your favored doneness.

Setting up the Gravy:

Coat a skillet with cooking oil and warmth at high setting. Blend in onions, mushrooms, and garlic. Whenever delicate, expel from the skillet and set it aside for a for a short time. Include the coconut flour into the skillet and blend in the coconut milk.

Keep blending at high warmth until the blend is smooth. Diminish the warmth when the blend is smooth and include the flavoring. Add the vegetable to the now practically thick sauce. Stew for another 5 to 10 minutes. Coat the cooked steaks with the thick sauce liberally and serve.

Paleo Pot Roast

Ingredients:

3 pounds rear end cook, with the fat cut
2 tbsp coconut oil
1 onion, enormous, chopped
2 celery ribs, cleaved
1/2 tbsp dried thyme
3 cloves garlic, minced
2 C hamburger soup (without additive)
1/2 tsp dried parsley
1 to 2 straight leaves
20 entire peppercorns
1/2 tbsp ocean salt
6 to 7 florets of cauliflower
2 carrots, cut
1/3 C coconut flour
1/2 tsp ocean salt

Directions:

Warmth coconut oil on a Dutch broiler or any thick-walled cooking pot. Include the back end broil and burn all sides. Expel the dish from the Dutch broiler and put it in a platter. Put the celery, parsley, onion, thyme, and garlic into the Dutch broiler and sauté for 5 minutes; Put the burned posterior meal back to the Dutch stove.

Include the stock, sound leaf, ocean salt and peppercorns. Spread and spot inside the broiler preheated to 3250 F. Cook the dish for 4 hours treating it each half hour. Evacuate broil after it is done and strain the stock into a bowl. Discard the vegetables keeping just the stock. Shred the meat with the utilization of two forks and put the destroyed meat again into the Dutch broiler.

Submerge the destroyed hamburger with the recently stressed fluid from the pot. Toss in the cauliflower, carrots and the rest of the ocean salt. Put inside the stove again and stew for an additional 45 minutes. Channel the stock from the Dutch broiler and measure. Include more hamburger juices on the off chance that important to make 3 cups of stock, at that point empty every one of the 3 cups into the pot. Mix in the flour and stew until it transforms into a thick sauce. Spread the meat and vegetables with the sauce.

Beef Roll

Ingredients:

1 ½ pound ground beef
1 egg
½ red or white onion (stripped and diced)
Dark pepper and salt to taste
½ tbsp olive oil
1/8 cup finely diced parsley

Directions:

Beat egg well in a little bowl and put in a safe spot. In a different bowl blend the ground hamburger with diced onion, pepper and salt. Include the egg into the meat blend and blend well. Fold parts of the meat blend into medium frankfurter sizes.

Line sauce skillet with olive oil and warmth at medium-high. Include each hamburger roll and flame broil until completely dark-colored everywhere. Expel the meat moves from the container and spot on a plate secured with a paper towel. Give it a chance to remain until the abundance fat channel. Organize the hamburger moves over your preferred vegetable. Brimming with new parsley drops and serve.

Shrimp, Cantaloupe and Mint Salad

Fixings:

3 C crisp Arugula
1 C ready mango solid shapes
crisp 1/2 lbs.
medium shrimps pre-cooked
3 tbsp Crisp lemon juice
1 Cup melon 3D squares
new 1 tsp nutmeg
1 tsp cinnamon

Directions:

Blend shrimp, melon, mango, nutmeg, cinnamon, and lemon juice. Top the plate of mixed greens blend with your decision of balsamic dressing. To set up the Balsamic Dressing: Combine olive oil, nectar and balsamic vinegar in a bowl. Serves 4

Paleo Grilled Salmon with Asparagus

Fixings:

1 lb salmon
1/2 lb cherry tomatoes
1/2 lb asparagus
1 tsp ocean salt
1 tbsp olive oil
1 tsp dark pepper

Fixings:

Line a skillet with olive oil and sauté until delicate the cut asparagus. Add pepper and salt to taste. Put in a safe spot while you set up the salmon. Clean crisp salmon and season as indicated by your taste. Sear salmon ensuring it is completely cooked start to finish. When cooked expel salmon from skillet and put in a safe spot. Spot the sautéed asparagus on a serving plate and spot the cooked salmon over it. Trimming with ½ lb cherry tomatoes and serve.

Paleo Chicken Stir Fry

Fixings:

1 lb boneless chicken cutlets
1/2 lb broccoli florets
5 cloves garlic finely cleaved
1/4 lb red ringer peppers (cut)
2 tbsp coconut oil
1/4 lb crisp carrots
1/4 lb finely cleaved chives
ocean salt and dark pepper to taste

Guidelines:

Put a little coconut oil to a fricasseeing and sauté chicken cutlets until seared and cooked altogether. Put the cooked chicken cutlets aside. Warmth coconut oil in another griddle. Include the broccoli, carrots, red pepper, garlic and chives. Stew until the vegetables are delicate. Include the chicken cutlets and season with pepper and salt to taste. Spot in a serving plate and serve.

Heated Chicken with Pomegranate Glaze

Ingredients:

1 entire chicken (around 4 to 5 lbs)
1 enormous lemon (punctured with fork)
1 tbsp Dijon mustard
2 sprigs rosemary, new
Seeds from 1 pomegranate
1 tbsp finely slashed garlic
2 sprigs crisp thyme
2 cups pomegranate juice, unsweetened 2 tbsp in addition to 1 tsp arrowroot
1 tsp nectar
1/2 ocean salt 1/2 tsp newly ground dark pepper

Directions:

Spot punctured lemon and rosemary inside the chicken hole. Tie the chicken legs together to keep it firm and set in a cooking skillet. Combine pomegranate juice, mustard, thyme, arrowroot, and garlic for treating. Pour the blend everywhere throughout the chicken and sprinkle with salt and pepper. Spot inside a stove preheated to 375 degrees. Prepare for 25 minutes. Take it out and season the chicken.

Prepare for an additional 25 minutes and afterward treat once more. Include the pomegranate seeds and diminish stove temperature to 350 degrees Fahrenheit.Bake for one more hour while seasoning each half hour this time. At the point when done deplete the fluid and put in a safe spot. Spread the chicken with foil and let represent 30 minutes. Serve the chicken with the coating.

Paleo Roasted Chicken and Herbal Gravy

Ingredients:

5 to 6 boneless chicken bosom (with skin)
1/2 tsp dried thyme
1 quart natural low sodium chicken juices
2 tbsp crisp rosemary (sprigs)
4 to 5 tbsp olive oil or coconut oil
8 squashed garlic cloves
2 to 3 tbsp coconut flour or almond flour.
ocean salt and pepper to taste

Directions:

Spread chicken bosoms with olive oil and season with pepper and salt. Mastermind in a preparing sheet that has been fixed with aluminum foil. Spot inside the broiler preheated to 350 degrees. Heat without spread until the chicken is totally cooked (around 30 minutes). Remove it from the broiler and cut the chicken bosoms on a level plane into 2 inch cuts.

For the Gravy

Warmth coconut oil in a sauce skillet over high warmth. Pour in the chicken stock, thyme, rosemary, salt, pepper and garlic. Blend well and steadily lessen warmth to low. Keep on stewing until you have the ideal surface and consistency. Spot cook chicken bosom, blend well, and afterward expel from flame. Serve hot.

Paleo Pumpkin and Chicken Curry

Ingredients:

2 pieces sliced chicken breasts
2 tablespoon olive oil
5 cups pumpkin, diced
2 garlic cloves, finely chopped
1 bunch fresh coriander
chopped 1 onion, diced
2 tbsp ginger, ground
1 tbsp turmeric, ground
2 tbsp coriander, ground
2 tbsp cumin, ground
1 ½ cups vegetable stock Salt

Instructions:

Sauté garlic and onion in a Fry pan for two minutes over medium heat.

Add chicken and simmer while stirring frequently for ten minutes until chicken turns white. Stir in the pumpkin, cumin, turmeric, ginger, and coriander and continue to stir for one minute. Pour the vegetable stock and simmer for 15minutes on low heat. Stir in the chopped coriander then put the cover on and simmer for another two minutes. Add salt to taste.

Egg and Capsicum Salad

Ingredients:

2 eggs, hard-boiled, diced
1tbsp coconut oil
2 diced bacon eyes
½ diced green capsicum
¼ C slashed parsley
1tbsp mayonnaise
1 C serving of mixed greens leaves, blended

Procedure:

Cook bacon in a coconut oil covered griddle over medium warmth. Broil the bacon until it begins to be fresh. Channel the abundance oil and move the bacon to a bowl. Include the bubbled eggs, parsley, capsicum, and mayonnaise. Hurl well. Orchestrate the plate of mixed greens on a serving plate and top with egg and capsicum blend to serve.

Prepared Chicken with Pomegranate Glaze

Ingredients:

1 entire chicken (around 4 to 5 lbs)
1 huge lemon (punctured with a fork)
1 tbsp Dijon mustard
2 sprigs rosemary, new
Seeds from 1 pomegranate
1 tbsp finely chopped garlic
2 sprigs new thyme
2 cups pomegranate juice unsweetened
2 tbsp in addition to 1 tsp arrowroot
1 tsp nectar
1/2 ocean salt
1/2 tsp newly ground dark pepper

Directions:

Spot punctured lemon and rosemary inside the chicken pit. Tie the chicken legs together to keep it firm and set in a simmering dish. Blend pomegranate juice, mustard, thyme, arrowroot, and garlic for seasoning. Pour the blend everywhere throughout the chicken and sprinkle with salt and pepper. Spot inside a stove preheated to 375 degrees. Heat for 25 minutes. Take it out and treat the chicken. Heat for an additional 25 minutes and afterward treat once more. Include the pomegranate seeds and diminish stove temperature to 350 degrees Fahrenheit. Heat for one more hour while treating each half hour this time. At the point when done deplete the fluid and put in a safe spot. Spread the chicken with foil and let represent 30 minutes. Serve the chicken with the coating.

Paleo Roasted Chicken and Herbal Gravy

Ingredients:

5 to 6 boneless chicken bosom (with skin)
1/2 tsp dried thyme
1-quart natural low sodium chicken stock
2 tbsp crisp rosemary (sprigs)
4 to 5 tbsp olive oil or coconut oil
8 squashed garlic cloves
2 to 3 tbsp coconut flour or almond flour.
Ocean salt and pepper to taste

Guidelines:

Spread chicken bosoms with olive oil and season with pepper and salt. Organize in a preparing sheet that has been fixed with aluminum foil. Spot inside the stove preheated to 350 degrees. Heat without spread until the chicken is cooked (around 30 minutes). Remove it from the stove and cut the chicken bosoms on a level plane into 2-inch cuts.

For the Gravy

Warmth coconut oil in a sauce container over high warmth. Pour in the chicken soup, thyme, rosemary, salt, pepper, and garlic. Blend well and progressively lessen warmth to low. Keep on stewing until you have the ideal surface and consistency. Spot broil chicken bosom, blend well, and after that expel from flame. Serve hot.

Paleo Pumpkin and Chicken Curry

Ingredients:

2 pieces cut chicken bosoms
2 tablespoon olive oil
5 cups pumpkin, diced
2 garlic cloves, finely cleaved
1 bundle new coriander,chopped
1 onion, diced
2 tbsp ginger, ground
1 tbsp turmeric, ground
2 tbsp coriander, ground
2 tbsp cumin, ground

1 ½ cups vegetable stock Salt

Guidelines:

Sauté garlic and onion in a Fry search for gold minutes over medium warmth. Include chicken and stew while blending regularly for ten minutes until chicken turns white. Blend in the pumpkin, cumin, turmeric, ginger, and coriander and keep on mixing for one moment. Pour the vegetable stock and stew for 15minutes on low warmth. Mix in the hacked coriander at that point put the spread on and stew for an additional two minutes. Add salt to taste.

Paleo Crispy Orange Chicken

Ingredients:

2 pounds chicken (deboned, skinless)
1/4 tsp pepper

1.5 tsp ocean salt

.5 Cup coconut feast/flour

1 tbsp coconut oil, additional virgin

1 egg

For the Glaze:

1 teaspoon garlic, minced

1 cup crisp squeezed orange

1.5 tsp ground orange skin

.5 C hoisin sauce

1/4 cup nectar

Dash of cayenne pepper Sea Salt Pepper

Guidelines:

Cut the chicken into two inch pieces and spot them in an enormous compartment or a blending bowl. Include the egg, coconut oil, pepper and ocean salt. Join well and set aside. Put the ½ cup coconut supper/flour blend in a different bowl and plunge the chicken on the flour blend ensuring each piece is covered liberally.

Get enough coconut oil to fill a big fry pan to about half an inch from its base. Put the fry pan on the stove and set the temperature on high warmth until it achieves 3750 F. Begin singing the chicken pieces by groups. Broil each cluster until the chicken cutlets are sautéed, fresh, and crunchy. This ought to be around 3-4 minutes for each cluster. Take out the chicken pieces from the skillet and channel them well over paper towels.

Wrap up the remainder of the chicken pieces and put them in a safe spot while you set up the coating. Expel all the oil from the skillet leaving just around 2 tbsp. of oil and lower the temperature to medium warmth.

Sauté the garlic for one moment however abstain from consuming it else it will give a harsh taste. Hurl in the various fixings and let the blend bubble. Blend the bubbling blend for three minutes before decreasing the warmth. Keep on stewing the blend until you produce the coating. Spread the chicken with the coating and enrich with chives and orange cuts before serving.

Stovetop Spring Frittata

Ingredients:

1 tablespoon olive oil
1 clove garlic minced
1 radish ground or finely cleaved
1/2 cup cleaved asparagus
3 eggs beaten
1 teaspoon crisp slashed mint
Ocean salt and crisp ground pepper to taste

Guidelines:
Warmth the oil in a little skillet over medium-low warmth. Include the garlic, radish, and asparagus and cook until relaxed. Season with salt and pepper. Include the eggs and cook for a moment until the edges are set. Lift the edges cautiously and let the fluid stream underneath the edges. Turn the warmth down to low and cover the container. Cook for 2-3 minutes until eggs are cooked through. Top with the crisp mint.

Egg and Capsicum Salad

Ingredients:

2 eggs, hard boiled, diced
1tbsp coconut oil
2 diced bacon eyes
½ diced green capsicum
¼ C slashed parsley
1tbsp mayonnaise
A cup serving of mixed greens leaves, blended

Guidelines:

Cook bacon in a coconut oil covered griddle over medium warmth. Broil the bacon until it begins to be firm. Channel the abundance oil and move the bacon to a bowl. Include the bubbled eggs, parsley, capsicum, and mayonnaise. Hurl well. Orchestrate the serving of mixed greens on a serving plate and top with egg and capsicum blend to serve.

Paleo bread recipes

Date and Walnut Bread

Ingredients:

½ C almond flour, whitened
2 tbsp coconut flour
¼ tsp heating soft drink
⅛ tsp celtic ocean salt
3 enormous Medjool dates
1 tbsp apple juice vinegar
3 eggs
½ cup pecans, slashed

Guidelines:

With a sustenance processor, blend almond flour and coconut flour and mix well together. Include preparing soft drink and salt. Heartbeat to mix. Include dates and heartbeat again until the blend has a similar surface as coarse sand. Mix in apple juice vinegar and eggs and mix well. Heartbeat in the pecans quickly. Pour the hitter on to a smaller than normal portion skillet. Put inside the broiler and heat for 28 to 32 minutes at 350° F. Cool the bread while still in search for gold hours before evacuating. Makes 1 little portion of Walnut Bread.

Dull Rye Bread

Ingredients:

1 cup almond flour, whitened
½ tsp baking soda
¾ tsp cream of tartar 3 eggs
2 tbsp olive oil
A ¼ cup of water
1 tsp nectar or nectar
1-2 tbsp caraway seeds

Directions:

Blend almond flour, flax, salt, heating soft drink and cream of tartar in an enormous bowl. In a different, littler bowl blend egg, oil, water, and agave. Mix in the dry fixings into wet. Include the caraway seeds and blend well. Let the player represent 1 to 2 minutes for it to thicken. Pour the player to a little, lubed portion container. Prepare for 30-35 minutes at 350° F.

Paleo Banana Bread

Ingredients:

1 ½ cups bananas (squashed)
1 tbsp nectar
1 tbsp vanilla concentrate
3 eggs
¼ Cup vegetarian shortening
½ tsp ocean salt
2 Cup almond flour, whitened
1 tsp heating soft drink

Guidelines:

Join bananas, nectar, vanilla, eggs, and shortening into the nourishment processor and heartbeat them together. Include the almond flour, heating soft drink, and salt while beating with every expansion. Empty the hitter into a recently lubed portion skillet . Prepare for 50 to an hour at 350°F. Remove from the broiler and cool before expelling from the container.

Cranberry Loaf Bread

Ingredients:

¾ C simmered almond spread, at room temperature
3 eggs
2 tbsp olive oil
¼ C arrowroot powder
¼ tsp heating soft drink
almond flour(blanched)
½ cup dried cranberries
olive oil
¼ Cup dried apricots(chopped)
¼ C sesame seeds
1 tsp ocean salt
¼ C sunflower seeds
¼ C pumpkin seeds
¼ cup in addition to
2 tbsp cut almonds

Guidelines:

Join the eggs, olive oil and almond spread in a huge bowl and mix until smooth utilizing a hand blender In a different medium size bowl, mix arrowroot powder, preparing soft drink and salt. Mix the wet blend with the arrowroot blend until all around blended. Crease in the cut almonds, dried apricots, sesame seeds, and cranberries.

Oil a portion container with olive oil and powder with almond flour. Move the hitter cautiously into the dish and top uniformly with whatever cut almonds left. Prepare for 40 to 50 minutes at 350° or until a blade embedded into focus tells the truth. Cool the bread for in any event 1 hour while in the skillet before evacuating.

PALEO SOUP RECIPES

Sopa de Lima

Ingredients:

4 parts chicken bosom
¼ tsp Chili Powder
4 Cups of Organic Chicken Broth (you can utilize your very own natively grown juices)
¼ tsp Garlic Powder.
2 pieces Chile Peppers
2 Tomatoes, sliced
4 to 5 Garlic Cloves, stripped and minced.
1 Tbsp Olive Oil
½ of an Onion, chopped
⅓ Cup Lime juice (or you can take the juice from 2 limes)
½ tsp Lime juice
2 Tbsp Cilantro, chopped
1 stripped Avocado, cleaved.
Ocean Salt

Guidelines:

Organize chicken in a preparing dish fixed with oil. Sprinkle the chicken with garlic and stew powder. Spot the heating dish inside the stove preheated to 400 degrees and prepare the Chicken for twenty minutes. Meanwhile, the chicken is preparing in the broiler, set a stock pot over the stove and include the olive oil. Sauté the Garlic, Onion and Serrano peppers together until they are delicate for three minutes. Mix in the Chopped Tomatoes and leave stewing for in any event two minutes more. Include lime juice and chicken stock while mixing once in a while. Alter temperature to low warmth. Expel the chicken from stove following two minutes and cool only enough for you to have the option to deal with it and hack it into little chomp sizes.

Return the slashed chicken pieces to the stock pot, and increment the warmth to carry the blend to bubble. When bubbling, bring down the warmth to the most minimal setting, and put on the top spread. Give it a chance to bubble daintily for an extra 20 minutes on low warmth. Spot the avocado pieces into each serving bowl (not legitimately into soup stock). Put the avocado in each bowl first at that point pour the soup over it. Wrap up by decorating with Cilantro.

Bacon Soup with Asparagus, Green Peas

Ingredients:

1 bundle asparagus, medium, cut

1/2 white onion, slashed
4 cups of bacon
3 Cup chicken stock (you can utilize vegetable stock as well)
2 cloves garlic, minced
1 C new peas (you can utilize solidified peas however defrost them first)
1/2 cup milk

Directions:

Utilize a wide-bottomed skillet to sear the bacon till they begin to be somewhat fresh. Expel them quickly from the skillet utilizing an opened spoon and set them aside to cool for some time. Disintegrate or Chop the bacon into minor pieces when cool enough. Sauté the onion and garlic utilizing a similar skillet till the onion turns brilliant. Include the peas and asparagus after. Stream in the chicken stock and let it bubble once more. Spread and lower the warmth. Permit to stew for twenty minutes before taking the skillet off the warmth. Utilize a hand-held blender to process the soup until it is smooth. Add flavoring as per taste. Top with bacon bits before serving.

Hot and Sour Chicken Soup

Ingredients:

2 tbsp Coconut Oil
1 Cup Onion, cut
1/2 Cup carrots, diced
1/2 Cup Celery, cut
2 Skinless Chicken Breast-medium diced
6 Cups Chicken Stock
5 Mushrooms, cut
1 tbsp crisp ginger minced
3 cloves garlic
3 tbsp Coconut Aminos
1/2 tsp Honey
3 tbsp White Wine Vinegar
1/2 tsp Sesame Oil
2 tbsp Tapioca Starch broke down in 0.5 cup chicken juices.
6 Eggs, beaten
2 Green Onions Chopped
1/2 Cup Bamboo Shoots meagerly Sliced Salt
Pepper
Hot Chili Oil

Guidelines:

Sauté onions in a substantial pot over medium/high warmth for 3 minutes. Include the carrots and cut onions. Keep on sauté until carrots become delicate. Pour in the chicken stock and hold up till it bubbles. Toss in the mushrooms, ginger, coconut oil, garlic, vinegar, nectar, and sesame oil in a specific order.

Increment the temperature to heat the blend to the point of boiling. Energetically whisk the custard starch with the chicken juices and empty in the custard arrangement into the stock pot with the soup while blending the soup persistently. Enable the soup to bubble once more. Keep on blending until the soup is thick at that point decrease the warmth to medium.

Sprinkle the whisked eggs gradually over the bubbling soup while mixing consistently. Include the green onions, bamboo shoots, pepper, and salt together with a modest quantity of the stew oil. Diminish the warmth to Low this time and let it stew for 5 minutes. Taste the soup. Include more bean stew oil if necessary only a little at any given moment until the taste is zesty enough for you.

Occasion Bouillabaisse

Fixings:

1 can diced tomatoes
28 oz crisp cleaved tomatoes
1 onion, medium, slashed
1 medium red ringer pepper
3 to 4 stalks celery, cut and slashed
2 cloves garlic, slashed
½ lb shelled medium shrimps, deveined
¼ lb. swordfish, cleaned and cut in blocks
½ lb. cove scallops
½ tsp cinnamon
1 tsp cumin
cayenne pepper
dark pepper and Salt
2 cups of water

Guidelines:

You ought to have around equivalent volumes of cleaved onions, chile peppers, and celery. Include in any if necessary. Sauté onion, garlic, ringer pepper, and celery, in 3 tablespoon olive oil. Include dark pepper and salt. Include the swordfish 3D shapes and keep on cooking until the vegetables are delicate yet firm. Include the tomatoes, two cups of water, cinnamon and cumin.

Put some of the cayenne pepper as per your preference. Heat it until it boils for five minutes. Include the shrimp and continue boiling the mixture for an additional 4 minutes. Mix in the scallops and keep boiling for one more moment this time. Lessen to low warmth. Close the lid of the container and permit to stew for at the very least 25 minutes and close to 30 minutes. Garnish with crisp parsley sprigs and serve.

PALEO DINNER RECIPES

Sheep Veggie Stew

Ingredients :

2 tablespoons olive oil
1 Onion cut
1 Carrot cut
1 Zucchini cut
1 Green pepper cut
1 teaspoon Italian flavoring
1 pound sheep cubed
4 cups Chicken juices
crisp cleaved parsley for serving

Guidelines:

Warmth the oil in an enormous soup pot. Include the vegetables and cook until mellowed. Include the Italian flavoring, and the sheep and cook until sheep are caramelized. Blend in the soup and heat to the point of boiling. Lessen warmth and stew until sheep are delicate. Serve beat with the hacked parsley.

Cooked Brussels Sprouts with Bacon

Ingredients

2 pounds Brussels sprouts divided
2 tablespoons olive oil
8 bacon cuts cooked and disintegrated
Ocean salt and new ground pepper to taste

Directions

Put the sprouts in steamer crate or microwave and steam until simply delicate. Evacuate and let cool marginally. Hurl the steamed sprouts with the olive oil and a spot of salt. Lay on a material lined preparing sheet, cut side up. Preheat grill to high warmth and cook until tops are all around caramelized. Hurl with the bacon and serve warm.

Balsamic Chicken Salad

Ingredients

Chicken
1/2 cup olive oil
1/4 cup Balsamic vinegar
1 teaspoon Dijon mustard
1/2 teaspoon ocean salt
1/4 teaspoon dark pepper

Salad
8 cups hacked Romaine lettuce
2 Large tomatoes quartered
2 cups cooked and hacked green beans
Juice of 2 lemons

1/4 cup olive oil

Directions

Whisk the olive oil, vinegar, and mustard in a little bowl with the salt and pepper. Brush half over the chicken bosoms. Preheat flame broil to medium-high warmth. Barbecue the chicken until cooked through, permit to cool and cut. Prepare the plate of mixed greens in a huge bowl with the lemon juice and olive oil and top with the cut chicken.

Chicken and Vegetable Bowl

Ingredients

3 tablespoons olive oil
2 cloves garlic minced
2 Bell peppers any shading, cut
1 Red onion cut
4 cups Spinach slashed
1/2 cup destroyed carrots
2 tablespoons Lemon juice
1/2 cup Chopped crisp parsley
2 cups cooked and destroyed chicken bosom
Sprouts for garnishing
Ocean salt and new ground pepper to taste

Directions

Warmth the oil in an overwhelming bottomed skillet over medium warmth. Include the garlic, peppers, and onion and cook until diminished. Include the spinach and carrots and cook until spinach is withered. Include the parsley and lemon squeeze and mood killer heat. Mix the chicken into the vegetables and serve beat with the sprouts.

Spring Lamb Stir Fry

Ingredients:

3 tablespoons Coconut oil
1 pound boneless sheep cubed
2 cloves garlic minced
1 teaspoon crisp ginger
2 Zucchini cut
1 enormous carrot cut
1 teaspoon Ground coriander
1 teaspoon Ground cumin
Juice of 1 lime
crisp cleaved cilantro
Cauliflower rice for serving
Ocean salt and crisp ground pepper to taste

Guidelines:

Warmth the coconut oil in an enormous skillet. Include the sheep and cook until sautéed. Expel from skillet and include the garlic, ginger, zucchini, and carrots. Cook until mellowed. Include the coriander, cumin, and lime squeeze, and add the sheep back to the container. Keep cooking until sheep is finished. Serve beat with the cilantro and with cauliflower rice.

Greek Chicken and Veggie Skewers

Ingredients:

Marinade
1/2 cup olive oil
2 lemons, squeezed
1 teaspoon Red wine vinegar
2 tablespoons Chopped crisp parsley
2 tablespoons cleaved new mint
1 teaspoon Oregano
1/2 teaspoon Sea salt
1/2 teaspoon Fresh ground dark pepper

Sticks
1.5 pounds boneless chicken cubed
1 half quart Cherry tomatoes
1 Red onion cubed
2 Zucchini cubed
1 half quart Button mushrooms

Instructions:

Mix the marinade ingredients in a container and mix them well. Wire the chicken and greens upon skewers and lay in a shallow dish. Spill the marinade over top. Cool for at least 3 hours, rolling occasionally. When set to cook, take out the skewers from the refrigerator and preheat a gas or charcoal grill to medium-high heat. Grill the skewers until rooster is cooked through and veggies are slightly browned.

Roasted Vegetables with Bacon

Ingredients:

4 cuts bacon slashed
1 onion cut
1 pound Brussel sprouts divided
1/2 pound little radishes divided
1/2 head broccoli cut into florets
ocean salt to taste
crisp ground dark pepper to taste

Guidelines:

Heat a big fry pan over medium-high flame. Include the bacon and cook until it gets crispy. Expel the bacon from the dish, leaving behind only the fat. Add the onion and cook until mellowed.First, cook the Brussel sprouts and cook them until they are lightly burned and then include the radishes and broccoli in them. Keep cooking them till the veggies are lightly burnt. In the end, add the bacon back to the skillet before you serve the meal.

Turkey Bowl with Kale and Sweet Potatoes

Ingredients:

3 cups Dinosaur kale (cut into nibble measured pieces)
2 cups Turkey bosom (cooked and cleaved)
1/4 cup Dried cranberries
1/4 cup Toasted sunflower seeds
1/4 cup olive oil
2 tbsp Cider vinegar
1 tbsp Dijon mustard
2 tbsp Real maple syrup
3 strips Cooked bacon (disintegrated)
2 Sweet potatoes (stripped and cubed)

Directions:

Put the sweet potatoes in a pot and spread it with virus water. Heat to the point of boiling and decrease warmth to a stew. Stew for 10 to 15 minutes, until delicate. Channel. Backrub the kale in an enormous bowl for a few minutes, until leaves are delicate and separated. Include the potatoes, cranberries, and sunflower seeds to the bowl. In a different bowl whisk the olive oil, juice vinegar, mustard, maple syrup, and salt and pepper until very much joined. Prepare it with the serving of mixed greens. Include the turkey and bacon before serving.

Paleo Italian Meatballs and Braised Greens

Ingredients:

2 tbsp olive oil
2 tbsp Italian flavoring
2 cloves garlic (minced)
1/4 cup Almond Flour
1 tsp Paprika
1/2 tsp Sea salt
1/2 lbs Ground hamburger
1 Onion (finely slashed)

Greens:

4 cuts bacon (diced)
1 bundle Collard greens (stems evacuated and cleaved)
1 bundle Swiss chard (stems evacuated and cleaved)
1 cup Chicken juices (or water)
2 tsp Apple juice vinegar
Ocean salt and crisp ground pepper

Guidelines:

Preheat broiler to 400 degrees Fahrenheit. Join the hamburger, onion, garlic, almond flour, paprika, and salt in a huge bowl. Utilizing your hands, blend until simply joined, being mindful so as not to over blend. Structure into 2-inch meatballs and lay on a heating sheet. Brush with the olive oil and coat with the Italian flavoring. Heat for 20-30 minutes, until cooked through. To make the greens, cook the bacon an enormous, profound skillet until it begins to darker. Add the greens and mix to coat in the fat. Add the soup or water to cover the greens and go down to low. Give the greens a chance to stew for around 10 minutes over low warmth until greens are delicate. Serve the meatballs over the greens.

Paleo Buffalo Mushroom Skewers

Ingredients:

1 pound Button mushrooms
1/2 cup Hot sauce
2 tbsp olive oil
1/2 tsp Sea salt

Directions:

With a paper towel, cautiously clean the mushrooms, yet don't get them wet. Leave entire, yet expel the stems whenever wanted. Whisk the hot sauce, olive oil, and salt in a bowl. Add the mushrooms and hurl to coat. To cook the mushrooms, string them on sticks and lay on a preparing sheet (or on the other hand, you can leave them off the sticks) Bake for 15 minutes in a 375-degree broiler, or flame broils them on a barbecue over medium-high warmth. Serve warm.

PALEO DESSERT RECIPES

Paleo chocolate chip treats

Ingredients:

1 egg, marginally beaten
1 teaspoon vanilla concentrate
1/4 cup coconut oil, softened and cooled
1/2 cup coconut sugar
1 cup almond flour
1/4 cup coconut flour
1/2 teaspoon heating soft drink

3 oz 80% dim chocolate, coarsely chopped*
Coarse ocean salt, for sprinkling

Guidelines:

Preheat broiler to 350 degrees Fahrenheit. In a big bowl add beaten egg, softened and cooled coconut oil, coconut sugar, and vanilla concentrate. Next include almond flour, coconut flour, and heating soft drink, blending great to consolidate and frame a batter. Crease in dull chocolate pieces. You may need to utilize your hands to saturate the batter with the goal that it sticks together well. Utilize a treat scoop or huge tablespoon to drop batter onto an ungreased preparing sheet. Tenderly smooth the batter with your hand. Prepare for 11-13 minutes, or until edges are marginally brilliant dark colored. Sprinkle with coarse ocean salt and permit to cool on the treated sheet for 10 minutes before moving to a wire rack to completing the process of cooling. Makes 12 treats.

Twofold chocolate hazelnut treats with sea salt

Ingredients:

2 cups crude hazelnuts
1 teaspoon coconut oil
1/4 teaspoon salt
2/3 cup coconut sugar
1/2 teaspoon vanilla concentrate
1 egg
1 egg yolk
1/2 cup great quality unsweetened cocoa powder
1 teaspoon baking soda
3 oz your preferred dull chocolate bar, slashed (in any event 72%, with no soy)
Coarse ocean salt, for sprinkling

Directions:

Preheat stove to 350 degrees F. Equally spread hazelnuts onto an enormous preparing sheet. Toast the hazelnuts in the stove for 8-10 minutes. Expel from the stove and let cool for 5-10 minutes. Keep heat in the stove. Move hazelnuts to the bowl of a nourishment processor and procedure for 10-15 minutes or until it transforms into a hazelnut spread; you'll likely need to scratch down the sides every now and again. We need this to be velvety so try to get it that way. When it begins to get velvety, include a teaspoon of coconut oil and the salt and procedure again for one more moment or two. Presently let the nut margarine sit for 5-10 minutes until it chills off a bit. This is significant so remember to do it! Else you'll finish up with a cooked egg. Include the coconut sugar, vanilla, egg, and additional egg yolk. Procedure again until all around joined and a batter starts to shape. Next include cocoa powder and baking soda, and procedure once more. The mixture may turn into an enormous ball, so if that happens simply move the batter to a medium bowl and utilize a wooden spoon to blend everything until all around joined. Next mix in slashed chocolate. Structure batter into 1/2 inch balls, place on treat sheet and level the mixture with the palm of your hand. I like to level mine quite dainty. Prepare for 8-10 minutes at that point expel from broiler and sprinkle with ocean salt. Enable treats to cool on the treat sheet for a couple of minutes before moving to a wire rack to cool totally. Makes around 18 treats

Paleo No Bake Cookie Dough Truffles

Ingredients:

½ tablespoon flaxseed seed
1 tablespoon unsweetened almond milk
2 tablespoons softened coconut oil
3 tablespoons coconut sugar
1 teaspoon vanilla concentrate
½ cup pressed almond flour
2 tablespoons coconut flour
⅛ teaspoon salt
1½ tablespoon dim chocolate chips, dairy free whenever wanted

For the chocolate covering:

⅓ cup dim chocolate chips, dairy free whenever wanted
1 teaspoon coconut oil

Directions:

In a medium bowl combine flaxseed dinner, almond milk, liquefied coconut oil, vanilla, and coconut sugar. In a little bowl combine almond flour, coconut flour, and salt. Gradually add the flour blend to the wet fixings. Blend well until a treat mixture consistency shapes. Crease chocolate chips into the treat mixture. Fold treat mixture into 1 tablespoon estimated balls, place on material lined preparing sheet and stop for 10 minutes. Following 10 minutes, soften the chocolate chips and coconut oil in a little pan over exceptionally low warmth, blending much of the time. You can likewise microwave the chocolate in a little microwave safe bowl in 20-second augmentations until softened. Rapidly utilize a fork to plunge every treat batter ball into the chocolate, trying to coat uniformly. Move back to material fixed preparing sheet and sprinkle with a little coarse ocean salt whenever wanted. Promptly spot heating sheet back in cooler for 20 minutes. Makes 8 treat mixture chomps. Keep in cooler until prepared to eat.

Paleo Banana Zucchini Muffins

Ingredients:

1 cup destroyed zucchini (from 1 medium zucchini)
1/2 cup squashed banana (from 1 medium banana)
3/4 cup cashew margarine
1/4 cup unadulterated maple syrup
2 eggs
1 teaspoon vanilla concentrate
1/2 cup coconut flour
1 teaspoon heating soft drink

1/4 teaspoon salt

Guidelines:

Preheat broiler to 350 degrees F. Line a biscuit tin with 10 biscuit liners. You're just making 10 biscuits, so forget two liners. Press destroyed zucchini of overabundance dampness with a paper towel. In a huge bowl, include zucchini, banana, cashew spread, maple syrup, eggs and vanilla. Blend until smooth and all around consolidated. Next add the dry fixings to the wet fixings: coconut flour, heating soft drink and salt. Blend until consolidated. Separation player equitably between 10 biscuit cups. Prepare for 22-27 minute or until toothpick confesses all and the highest points of the biscuits are simply marginally brilliant dark colored. Makes 10 biscuits.

CHAPTER 12

CONCLUSION AND PROPOSAL

I assume that this fashion is worth giving an attempt to seeing for yourself if you'll be able to comply with this lifestyle or not. One amongst the main issue that this fashion has extremely done is that it's helped heaps of individuals with their weight and health connected problems particularly and folks usually have seen their bodies remodeling from corpulent to slim and lean and it's one of the good virtues of the Paleo diet and one of the main attraction of this diet style and if paleo diet has worked for those people then it can even work for you,but it all depends on you whether or not you would like to give it an attempt or not. however, with thereupon they are also are other things to stay in mind whereas considering beginning the Paleo diet:
What level of processed food is suitable to you, by that term I mean the food that's changed in a way like canned goods, etc. you've got to see what level of processed food you're able to incorporate in your diet plan. there's no proper way to certify what Paleo diet is, therefore, this generally gets confusing for folks to outline what Paleo is, therefore, you would like to try and do your analysis furthermore to seek out what you actually ascertain Paleo diet to be for yourself and incorporate that diet set up in your lifestyle. You would have to rule out the skepticism within the validity of Paleo and therefore to try and do that you just got to verify what folks consider Paleo collectively to rule out ambiguity.
The end to all the discussion above is that the message is unbelievably obvious which is that the modern western eating routine that comprises of high and high carb nourishments isn't getting the opportunity to work for your well being and shape inside the long run and you would need to change over back to the sustenances that are suitable for the figure along these lines you have to ask yourself instructed as far as Paleo diet and join in your life though for a short amount of your opportunity to look at anyway the outcomes commencement to be and on the off chance that get happy with the consequence of this eating regimen set up, at that point voila you've discovered the enchantment key to great well being and readiness for an amazing remainder. Along these lines, at last, all I ask of you is to give this eating regimen plan a month's time and that I am very positive that in the event that you pursue this eating regimen plan for a month's time you'll probably not be coming back to the high sugar, high sodium diet that we are accustomed to having by and by. So I wish you a glad Paleo and good luck for what's to come.